The Own-Children Method

of Fertility Estimation

The Own-Children Method
of Fertility Estimation

LEE-JAY CHO
ROBERT D. RETHERFORD
MINJA KIM CHOE

An East–West Center Book
from the Population Institute

Library of Congress Cataloging-in-Publication Data

Cho, Lee-Jay.
   The own-children method of fertility estimation.

   "An East-West Center book."
   Bibliography: p.
   1.   Fertility, Human—Statistical methods.
I.   Retherford, Robert D.   II.   Choe, Minja Kim, 1941–
III.   Title.
HB901.C49   1986   304.6'32   86–19677
ISBN 0–86638–082–5

Distributed by University of Hawaii Press:
Order Department
University of Hawaii Press
2840 Kolowalu Street
Honolulu, Hawaii 96822

*This book is dedicated to the
national statistics bureaus and offices
of Asia and the Pacific*

CONTENTS

LIST OF FIGURES

LIST OF TABLES

LISTINGS OF COMPUTER PROGRAMS

PREFACE

It is now more than two decades since the own-children method of fertility estimation was first developed and applied to census data to obtain estimates of differential fertility for the United States. Early applications of the method involved simple calculations of age-specific birth rates based on child–woman ratios. Since then the method has undergone several refinements, and extensions have been developed to estimate age-specific marital birth rates, duration-specific ever-marital birth rates (with duration measured since first marriage), age–parity-specific birth rates and birth probabilities, and age-specific birth rates for men. The method has been used not only to obtain fertility estimates by characteristics, the principal application in more developed countries, but also to obtain basic estimates of age-specific birth rates and total fertility rates in less developed countries where birth registration is unreliable. Thus the own-children method has become a standard tool in the demographer's repertoire of indirect fertility estimation techniques. The method has been applied most extensively in Asia (including China), Latin America, and the United States. It has also been applied in Africa and Europe.

Publications reporting on the various methodological refinements and applications are numerous and scattered, and some of the documentation presented here has never been published. The purpose of this volume is to synthesize this earlier work into a single document in order to render the methodology more accessible and convenient to users.

Many colleagues contributed directly or indirectly to the development of this book. The early development of the method owes much to the late Wilson H. Grabill. William Brass provided encouragement and valuable technical advice leading to several refinements. We are also grateful to Ansley J. Coale for his helpful comments and encouragement. We are especially grateful to our coauthors of previous research papers and reports, which, with their kind permission, are drawn on freely throughout. Additional thanks are due to Griffith Feeney, who over the years has made numerous helpful suggestions, particularly on how to incorporate indirect methods of mortality estimation into the methodology. The extension of the method to estimate birth rates by age and duration since first marriage for ever married women grew out of a suggestion from Charles F. Westoff. Victoria Ho, Ruby Bussen, Ann Midkiff, Judith Ann L. Tom, and the late Howard Brunsman all made major contributions to developing computer programs for applications. Robin Loomis provided valuable research assistance in the preparation of tables and graphics. We are also grateful to Kenneth Hill, who read the entire manuscript and suggested many improvements. Grants from the U.S. Agency for International Development and the U.S. Bureau of the Census supported much of the research leading to this book. The preparation of the book itself was supported by a grant from the Ford Foundation. Finally, we are indebted to the national statistics bureaus and offices in the Asian and Pacific region for their cooperation, contributions, and efforts in applying the own-children method to census and survey data and in publishing the results.

CHAPTER I

Introduction

In most nations birth registration is incomplete and conventional measurement of fertility from vital statistics is difficult or impossible. Many of these nations, however, have for some time routinely conducted population censuses and surveys. By applying indirect demographic estimation techniques, demographers have been able to use census and survey data to fill many of the gaps in our knowledge of fertility levels and trends. Some of these techniques, including the own-children method, have the additional capability of producing fertility estimates by social and economic characteristics asked about in censuses or surveys. This feature makes the indirect methods useful even in situations in which vital registration is virtually complete, since information on social and economic characteristics is not usually recorded on birth certificates. Consequently, many of the indirect estimation techniques originally developed for situations in which vital registration was seriously deficient will remain useful even as vital registration improves.

The own-children method in brief

The own-children method of fertility estimation is a reverse-survival technique for estimating age-specific birth rates for years previous to a census or household survey. From the basic household records, on computer tape or in other machine-readable form, enumerated children are first matched to mothers within households, usually on the basis of answers to questions on age, sex, marital status, number of living children, and relation to head of household. Sometimes matching is facilitated by a special census question on line number (in the household listing) of mother, if present. In either case, a computer algorithm is used for matching. The matched (i.e., own) children, classified by their own ages and mother's age, are then reverse-survived to estimate numbers of births by age of mother in previous years. Reverse-survival is similarly used to estimate numbers of women by age in previous years. After adjustments are made for misenumeration (mainly undercount and age misreporting) and unmatched (i.e., non-own) children, age-specific birth rates are calculated by dividing the number of reverse-survived births by the number of reverse-survived women. Estimates are normally computed for each of the fifteen years or groups of years before the census. Estimates are not usually computed further back than fifteen years because births must then be based on children aged 15 or more at enumeration, a large proportion of whom do not reside in the same household as their mother and hence cannot be matched. (If marriage is late and households are stable, however, twenty years of estimates are sometimes possible.) All calculations are done initially by single years of age and time. Estimates for grouped ages or calendar years are obtained by appropriately aggregating single-year numerators (births) and denominators (women) and then dividing the aggregated numerator by the aggregated denominator. Such aggregation is often useful for minimizing the distorting effects of age misreporting on the fertility estimates.

The basic logic of the procedure is illustrated by the simplified reverse-survival diagram in Figure 1.1. We suppose a census in 1970. $C_{3,27}$ denotes the number of children aged 3 who are matched to women aged

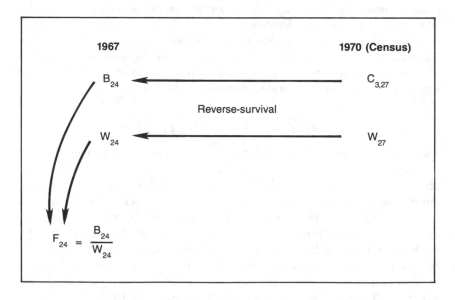

Figure 1.1. Reverse-survival diagram for own-children analysis

27 at the time of the census; we imagine that $C_{3,27}$ is already adjusted for undercount, age misreporting, and the presence of non-own (unmatched) children. W_{27} denotes the number of women aged 27 enumerated in the census; we similarly imagine that W_{27} is already adjusted for undercount and age misreporting. Three years ago the children, $C_{3,27}$, were births, B_{24}, to women aged 24, W_{24}. Because of intervening deaths, B_{24} is somewhat larger than $C_{3,27}$, and W_{24} is somewhat larger than W_{27}. The age-specific birth rate three years ago, F_{24}, is calculated as B_{24}/W_{24}.

Starting from this simple logic, the own-children method has undergone many refinements and elaborations over more than two decades of applications, described and summarized in the chapters that follow.

Historical development

The own-children method of fertility estimation originated in a series of special tabulations of young children by age of mother from the 1910 and 1940 censuses of the United States (U.S. Bureau of the Census 1947), which were used to generate estimates of differential fertility. Employing such tabulations, Wilson H. Grabill and Lee-Jay Cho developed the basic ideas of the method in the early 1960s (Grabill and Cho 1965). Further work occurred in a study of differential fertility in the United States (Cho, Grabill, and Bogue 1970). Cho (1971c) subsequently refined the approach to obtain annual fertility estimates for each of the ten years immediately preceding a census. The 1970 round of censuses ushered in applications of the method in countries around the world, including Bolivia, Brazil, Colombia, Costa Rica, Guatemala, Hungary, Indonesia, Japan, the Republic of Korea, Malaysia, Pakistan, Paraguay, the Philippines, and Thailand. (References to these studies are included in the bibliography at the end of this book.)

As the method was applied to more censuses, further refinements were made to handle problems such as age misreporting and changes in mortality levels during the past. For application in countries lacking reliable information on mortality from vital registration, the Brass method of estimating infant and child mortality (Brass 1975) and Feeney's extension of Brass's method, allowing for changing mortality (Feeney 1980) were incorporated into the procedure. A package of computer programs in three stages was developed.

More recent extensions of the own-children method include estimation of age–parity-specific birth rates (Retherford and Cho 1978), age-specific birth rates for currently married women (Ratnayake, Retherford, and Sivasubramaniam 1984), birth rates by age and duration since first marriage for ever-married women (Cho and Retherford 1978; Retherford, Cho, and Kim 1984), and age-specific birth rates for men (Retherford and Sewell 1986).

A promising new development, now being tested, involves the reconstruction of birth histories from data on own children. A woman and her own children represent a partial birth history. Omitted are deceased children, children living elsewhere, and children of ages 15 and older. The total number of births excluded equals the number of children ever born to the woman less the number of her own children. By considering the age of the woman, the birth dates of her own children, the number of excluded births, and the shape of the aggregate age-specific fertility schedule, it is possible to impute the birth dates of the excluded children and hence to arrive at a complete, reconstructed (though partially estimated) birth history for every woman. Although these reconstructed histories generally are not accurate at the individual level, preliminary tests indicate that the imputation can be carried out in such a way that they produce fertility statistics that are reasonably accurate at the aggregate level. When mortality is low and families are intact, the proportion of births that need to be imputed is quite small, so that even a rather crude imputation procedure should provide good results. Birth history data are essential for many kinds of fertility analysis, but they have thus far been available only from relatively small fertility surveys. The ability to reconstruct statistically valid birth history data from censuses and large-scale household surveys promises to open vast new areas for fertility research.

Strengths and limitations

The own-children method has several strengths. First, the method is useful in less developed countries where vital registration often is seriously deficient. In these countries, censuses as well as vital registration tend to suffer from undercount; but censuses, to which the own-children method can be applied, tend to be more accurate. Moreover, if omissions in censuses tend to be of entire households, then age-specific child–woman ratios tend to be biased comparatively little by undercount. Then own-children estimates of age-specific birth rates, which can be viewed as mortality-adjusted, age-specific child–woman ratios, also tend to be biased comparatively little by undercount.

A second strength is that own-children estimates of fertility can be tabulated by whatever characteristics are recorded in the census or household survey. This makes it possible, for example, to tabulate fertility estimates by such variables as education, occupation, language, and religion. Since vital registration systems do not normally collect information on these variables, fertility estimates derived from vital registration cannot be so tabulated. This feature of the own-children method makes it attractive in more developed as well as in less developed countries (see, for example, Cho, Grabill, and Bogue 1970; Rindfuss and Sweet 1977; Sweet and Rindfuss 1983).

A third strength is that the own-children method ordinarily requires no new data collection and is therefore inexpensive to apply. The typical application is to a census or household survey already undertaken for other purposes. Examples of suitable household surveys are labor force surveys and income and expenditure surveys. The only requirements are that the census or survey be of households, so that children may be matched to mothers within the same household, and that basic information on age and sex of respondents be asked. Ideally, additional information on marital status, number of children ever born or still living, and relationship to head of household should also be present, to facilitate matching, but in most instances satisfactory if slightly less accurate results can be obtained even when this supplemental information is missing.

A fourth strength relates to the large size of the census or household survey samples to which the own-children method is typically applied, relative to the small sample size of the typical fertility survey. Fertility surveys that collect maternity histories are usually based on a few thousand interviews and do not offer much potential for detailed cross-tabulation of fertility estimates for geographic subdivisions and by socioeconomic characteristics. In contrast, the census samples to which the own-children method is typically applied often contain upward of one million individuals, thereby providing a great deal of potential for cross-tabulation.

A fifth strength is that the own-children estimates of age-specific birth rates derived for each year during the fifteen-year estimation period immediately preceding the census or survey do not suffer from age truncation. This advantage stems from the fact that the initial matching of children to mothers is done for women up to age 65 at the time of enumeration. Fifteen years previous to enumeration these 65-year-old women were 50 years old. Therefore, age-specific birth rates can be calculated up to age 50 for each calendar year back to the fifteenth year before enumeration. Fertility estimates derived from maternity histories, on the other hand, suffer from age truncation. Typically, maternity histories are collected only from ever-married women aged 15–49. This means, for example, that age-specific birth rates can be calculated up to age 45 for the fifth year preceding the survey, age 40 for the tenth year preceding the survey, and age 35 for the fifteenth year preceding the survey. Thus maternity history data do not ordinarily allow a complete reconstruction of age-specific fertility in previous years.

The major limitation of the own-children method is that both the age pattern of fertility and the estimated trend of fertility can be severely distorted by age misreporting. Such distortions can be lessened but usually not eliminated by aggregating estimates over several calendar years. However, if the method is applied to two or more successive censuses, the estimated fertility trends for single calendar years partly overlap, since each census yields estimates for a fifteen-year period. For example, own-children fertility estimates derived from two censuses ten years apart yield trends that overlap during the first five years preceding the first census. The degree to which these two trends coincide during this five-year period may indicate the nature of systematic biases due to age misreporting, and the trend accordingly adjusted. Of course, sensitivity to age misreporting also characterizes fertility estimates derived from maternity histories. But, as we shall see later, the distortions due to age misreporting tend to be less pronounced in maternity histories because of differences in the way that data are collected.

A second limitation is that the own-children estimates may be biased by migration, although this is not usually much of a problem since migrants are normally a small proportion of a population. If migration rates are high, however, and if migrants are a highly selected group by virtue of their age-specific fertility behavior, then bias in the fertility estimates from this source can also be serious. For example, in instances of high rates of rural-to-urban migration, own-children estimates of fertility for urban areas in years before the survey tend to be too high because many of the urbanites interviewed at the time of the census lived a few years before in rural areas, where their fertility was much higher. On the other hand, if, in a particular geographic area, in-migrants have the same age-specific birth rates as nonmigrants, there is no bias from in-migration, unless some of the in-migrants leave their children with relatives in other geographic areas for long periods of time before becoming permanently resettled in the geographic area under consideration. Rather similar remarks pertain to potential biases introduced by out-migration. Fertility estimates derived from maternity histories also suffer from migration bias, although not in precisely the same way.

A third limitation is that the own-children method in its current state of development does not yield birth interval statistics. This deficiency exists because the household roster of surviving children who are matched to a particular woman does not yield a complete birth history. Given the ages of the surviving children matched to a woman, one can infer birth dates, yielding a partial birth history that omits births of children who later died or moved out of the household before being enumerated in the census. As mentioned earlier, however, it is possible to use probability models to impute the birth dates of the missing children and thereby reconstruct the complete birth history, provided that the census includes questions on number of children ever born and number of children still living. Preliminary tests indicate that aggregate-level birth interval statistics from birth histories reconstructed in this way compare quite well with those derived from maternity histories. This extension of the own-children method, which is still under development, clarifies why age misreporting and, to a lesser extent, migration tend to bias fertility estimates derived from own children and maternity histories in much the same way. Indeed, fertility estimates derived from own children can be viewed as fertility estimates derived from incomplete maternity histories.

A fourth limitation is that matching errors and misallocation of non-own children may introduce bias. But bias from these sources tends to be small compared with bias from age misreporting.

Purpose and organization of this book

The purpose of this book is twofold. The first is to provide a concise summary of the own-children methodology and problems of application. The second is to spell out step-by-step procedures for applying the methodology.

Chapter 2 outlines the basic methodology. Chapter 3 discusses major methodological extensions. Chapter 4 deals with evaluation and analysis of errors. Chapter 5 contains illustrative analyses for the Republic of Korea and Pakistan. Chapter 6 analyzes fertility trends estimated alternatively from birth histories and own-children data. Chapter 7 outlines step-by-step procedures for application, with illustrative examples. The appendices discuss specialized aspects of the method and selected computer programs.

CHAPTER 2

Basic Methodology

This chapter explains the core methodology for estimating age-specific birth rates. Although the methodology can be applied to household surveys as well as to censuses, in the interest of concision we discuss only censuses. The explanation of methodology is framed first in terms of continuous functions, then more realistically in terms of discrete functions.

Continuous formulation

The logic of the own-children method is most easily explained if age-specific birth rates, age distributions, and life table variables are viewed as continuous functions (Retherford, Cho, and Kim 1984). Let

$f_a(t)$: Instantaneous age-specific birth rate for women aged a at time t

$C_{x,a}$: Number of own children aged x of mothers aged a enumerated in the census

$B_a(t)$: Number of births to women aged a at time t

$W_a(t)$: Number of women aged a at time t

ℓ_y : Probability of surviving from birth to age y

ℓ_y^f : Probability of surviving from birth to age y for females.

The values of ℓ_y and ℓ_y^f are obtained from appropriate life tables for the population. In the continuous formulation, ages and times are conceptualized as exact ages and times rather than single-year age groups or time periods. (Note that, strictly speaking, $C_{x,a}$, $B_a(t)$, and $W_a(t)$ are density functions, defined as the number of persons per year of age or time.)

For simplicity we consider that numbers of women and children at the time of the census have already been adjusted for underenumeration, age misreporting, and the presence of unmatched (non-own) children, and that mortality has been constant over the estimation period. Then, with t denoting the time of the census,

$$B_{a-x}(t - x) = C_{x,a} (\ell_0/\ell_x) \tag{2.1}$$

$$W_{a-x}(t - x) = W_a(t) (\ell^f_{a-x}/\ell^f_a) \tag{2.2}$$

$$f_{a-x}(t - x) = B_{a-x}(t - x)/W_{a-x}(t - x). \tag{2.3}$$

Formula (2.1) reverse-survives children aged x of mothers aged a at time t to births of mothers aged $a - x$ at time $t - x$. Formula (2.2) reverse-survives women aged a at time t to women aged $a - x$ at time $t - x$.

Note that the age associated with an own-children estimate of an age-specific birth rate is the age obtaining at the time of childbirth, not at the time of the census. When the own-children estimates of fertility are tabulated by other characteristics such as education, however, these other characteristics normally pertain to the time of the census.

Discrete formulation

The actual computation of own-children fertility estimates is done with discrete age and time intervals. The base calculations are all done by single years of age and time (Retherford and Cho 1978:569–70). We have the following definitions:

$F_a(t)$: Single-year central age-specific birth rate for women aged a to $a + 1$ during calendar year t to $t + 1$

C_x : Number of children aged x to $x + 1$ enumerated in the census

$C_{x,a}$: Number of own children aged x to $x + 1$ of mothers aged a to $a + 1$ enumerated in the census

$B_a(t)$: Births during the period t to $t + 1$ to women aged a to $a + 1$ at time t

$W_a(t)$: Number of women aged a to $a + 1$ at time t

U^c_x : Adjustment factor for underenumeration and age misreporting of children aged x to $x + 1$

$U^c_{x,a}$: Adjustment factor for underenumeration and age misreporting of children aged x to $x + 1$ of mothers aged a to $a + 1$

U_a^w : Adjustment factor for underenumeration and age misreporting of women aged a to $a + 1$

V_x : Adjustment factor for non-own (unmatched) children, computed as the reciprocal of the proportion of children aged x to $x + 1$ at the time of the census who are matched to mothers

$R_{a \leftarrow b}$: Reverse-survival factor, from age group b to $b + 1$ to age group a to $a + 1$, for both sexes. If mortality has been constant over the estimation period, $R_{a \leftarrow b} = L_a/L_b$, where L_a denotes life table person-years lived between exact ages a and $a + 1$. If mortality has been changing, then

$$R_{a \leftarrow b} = \prod_{u=1}^{b-a} [L_{b-u}(t - u)/L_{b-u+1}(t - u)], \text{ where } L(t) \text{ is}$$

taken from the period life table for year t to $t + 1$. $R_{a \leftarrow b}^f$ denotes the reverse-survival factor for females only.

$r_{a \leftarrow b}$: Reverse-survival factor, from age group b to $b + 1$ to exact age a, for both sexes. If mortality has been constant over the estimation period, $r_{a \leftarrow b} = \ell_a/L_b$, where ℓ_a denotes the life table probability of surviving from birth to exact age a. If mortality has been changing, then

$$r_{a \leftarrow b} = [\ell_a(t - b + a - 1)/L_a(t - b + a - 1)]$$

$$\prod_{u=1}^{b-a} [L_{b-u}(t - u)/L_{b-u+1}(t - u)] \text{ if } a < b,$$

and $r_{a \leftarrow b} = \ell_a(t - 1)/L_a(t - 1)$ if $a = b$.

The calculation of central age-specific birth rates is illustrated in Figure 2.1. (Central, or age–period, rates pertain to squares or rectangles in the Lexis diagram shown in the figure.) Variable mortality and adjustments for underenumeration and age misreporting and for non-own children are now taken explicitly into account. For census enumeration at time t we have first that

$$B_a(t - x - 1) = C_{x,a+x+1} U_{x,a+x+1}^c V_x r_{0 \leftarrow x}, \tag{2.4}$$

corresponding to events in parallelogram CD, and that

$$W_a(t - x - 1) = W_{a+x+1}(t) U_{a+x+1}^w R_{a \leftarrow a+x+1}^f, \tag{2.5}$$

corresponding to the left edge of square BC. Then, by the logic of Figure 2.1,

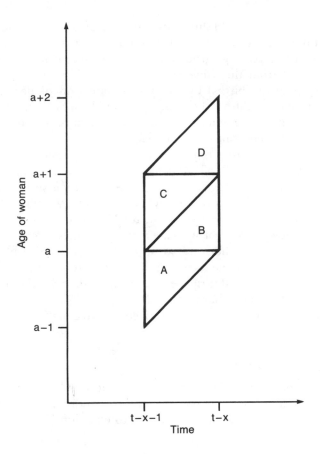

Figure 2.1. Lexis diagram for visualizing the calculation of $F_a(t - x - 1)$

Source: Retherford and Cho (1978:570).

Note: Births in the square BC are obtained by adding half of the births in AB to half of the births in CD. The midyear population in BC is likewise obtained by averaging the population at the beginning and end of the year, as represented by the left and right edges of the square BC. The symbol t denotes the time of the census and x denotes child's age.

$$F_a(t - x - 1) = [B_{a-1}(t - x - 1) + B_a(t - x - 1)]/[W_a(t - x - 1) + W_a(t - x)]. \tag{2.6}$$

This rate corresponds to births in square BC divided by the midyear number of women in square BC. On the right-hand side of (2.6), numerator and denominator are each obtained by an averaging procedure, as indicated in Figure 2.1. Multiplicative factors of 0.5 in the numerator and denominator cancel in the quotient and are not shown. Age-specific birth rates in five-year age groups over one or more calendar years are easily obtained from the single-year rates by dividing the appropriate sum of numerators (births) by the appropriate sum of denominators (women) from the right-hand side of equation (2.6). Such aggregation is particularly useful for minimizing errors from age misreporting in applications where the reporting of ages is inaccurate.

The adjustment factors require additional explanation (Retherford, Choe, and Wanglee 1978). The factors U_x^c and U_a^w are normally obtained from an indpendent source, such as a postenumeration survey. The factor $U_{x,a}^c$ is derived in the following way: First, because we adjust the number of women aged a to $a + 1$ by the factor U_a^w, we adjust the number of own children aged x to $x + 1$ who are matched to these women, $C_{x,a}$, by the same factor. At the same time we adjust the total number of children aged x to $x + 1$, C_x, by the factor U_x^c. These two requirements together imply that the overall adjustment factor, $U_{x,a}^c$, for own children, $C_{x,a}$, should be proportional to both U_a^w and U_x^c.

These considerations can be summarized by two equations,

$$U_{x,a}^c = k_x U_a^w U_x^c \tag{2.7}$$

$$U_x^c C_x = \Sigma_a(U_{x,a}^c V_x C_{x,a}), \tag{2.8}$$

where k_x is a proportionality factor, shown below to be a function of x, and V_x is the adjustment factor for non-own children. Substituting the expression for $U_{x,a}^c$ from equation (2.7) into equation (2.8) and solving for k_x, we obtain

$$k_x = C_x/[V_x\Sigma_a(U_a^w C_{x,a})], \tag{2.9}$$

which establishes that k_x is indeed a function of x. Substituting this expression for k_x back into equation (2.7) we obtain

$$U_{x,a}^c = (U_a^w U_x^c C_x)/[V_x\Sigma_a(U_a^w C_{x,a})]. \tag{2.10}$$

Since $C_x = \Sigma_a(V_x C_{x,a})$, equation (2.10) may be rewritten as

$$U_{x,a}^c = (U_a^w U_x^c \Sigma_a C_{x,a})/(\Sigma_a U_a^w C_{x,a}). \tag{2.11}$$

Values of $U_{x,a}^c$ are derived in practice from equation (2.11). In many instances, of course, no postenumeration survey is available. Then equation (2.11) cannot be applied, and $U_{x,a}^c$ and U_a^w are simply set to one.

In applications of the own-children method, years previous to the census are demarcated in twelve-month intervals starting with the census date. For example, for a census taken with a reference date of 1 November 1980, the year before the census extends from 1 November 1979 to 31 October 1980, which is not a normal calendar year starting on 1 January. The convention for labeling these offset calendar years is the following: Since, in this example, more than half of the year before the census occurs in calendar year 1980, the year before the census is labeled 1980. Had the census been taken on 1 April instead of 1 November 1980, then more than half of the year before the census would fall in calendar year 1979 and the year before the census would then have been labeled 1979. If desired, rates for offset calendar years can be interpolated linearly to standard calendar years extending from 1 January to 1 January. Normally this is done only when one wishes to compare precisely fertility estimates derived by the own-children method with estimates derived from vital registration. Henceforth we shall refer frequently to years of time as calendar years, even when they do not run from 1 January to 1 January.

Illustrative results for Sri Lanka

Figure 2.2 provides a simple illustration of one of the graphical formats in which final estimates are typically presented. In this case the application was to the 1981 Census of Sri Lanka (Ratnayake, Retherford, and Sivasubramaniam 1984). The data consisted of a 10 percent sample, including approximately 1.4 million individuals, created by selecting systematically every tenth census block from the full count. The large sample size allowed detailed cross-tabulations of the fertility estimates, illustrated in Figure 2.2 with a cross-tabulation of trends in total fertility by education and urban–rural residence. In this case, the detailed own-children estimates of age-specific birth rates by education and residence were aggregated to total fertility rates (TFRs), calculated by summing age-specific birth rates in five-year age groups and multiplying the sum by five. Summary measures such as the TFR are useful for reducing the mass of detailed age-specific fertility estimates to readable proportions.

Supplementary options

Period-cohort rates. In most applications of the own-children method, age–period (or central) age-specific birth rates are calculated, corresponding in the single-year case to squares in the Lexis diagram. It is also possible to calculate what have come to be called period–cohort rates, pertaining to parallelograms such as parallelogram CD in the Lexis diagram in Figure 2.1. Denoting period–cohort rates by $F_a^*(t)$, we have that

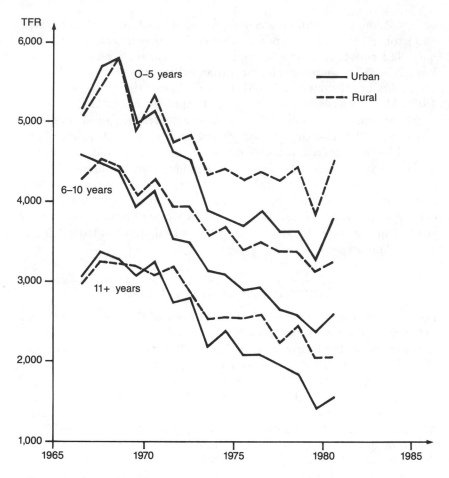

Figure 2.2. Own-children estimates of total fertility rates, by completed years of education and urban–rural residence, derived from the 1981 Census: Sri Lanka, 1966–80

Source: Ratnayake, Retherford, and Sivasubramaniam (1984:24).

Note: Throughout this book, rates and probabilities are expressed on a per-thousand basis.

$$F_a^*(t - x - 1) = B_a(t - x - 1)/\{.5[W_a(t - x - 1) \\ + W_{a+1}(t - x)]\} \tag{2.12}$$

where the B's and W's on the right-hand side of (2.12) are obtained from equations (2.4) and (2.5). The age subscript and the time argument of F^* in (2.14) denote age and time at the earliest time point in the parallelogram. Thus $F_a^*(t)$ pertains to fertility during the period t to $t + 1$ for women aged a to $a + 1$ at the beginning of the period.

If the own-children method is applied to a series of censuses, the period–cohort age-specific birth rates may be chained together along cohort corridors in the Lexis diagram to reconstruct the entire age-specific fertility experience of real cohorts.

Interpolation of life tables. The reverse-survival procedure assumes that complete life tables by sex and single years of age are available for each of the fifteen years preceding the census. Often this is not the case. Typically life tables are available only for some years (usually census years) and are abridged to age groups 0, 1–4, 5–9, 10–14, etc. In this situation the available period life tables must be interpolated to single years of time and age. First, linear interpolation (and, if necessary, extrapolation) of the initial abridged period life tables is performed on the $_nq_x$ (life table probability of dying between ages x and $x + n$) values of these tables to yield interpolated $_nq_x$ values for the midpoints of other calendar years or groups of calendar years within the estimation period. Period life table values of ℓ_x (survivors) at abridged ages are then computed for each of these other calendar years as $\ell_{x+n} = \ell_x(1 - {}_nq_x)$. Values of L_0 and L_{85+} (person-years of exposure at age 0 and at ages 85 and over) are also linearly interpolated for these other years.

The precise procedure for interpolation or extrapolation from initial period life tables for calendar years t_1 and t_2 is as follows: Suppose the quantity to be interpolated is $_nq_x$. Assume that the $_nq_x$ changes linearly over time. Then for any time t,

$$_nq_x(t) = {}_nq_x(t_1) + [(t - t_1)/(t_2 - t_1)][{}_nq_x(t_2) - {}_nq_x(t_1)]. \tag{2.13}$$

Although linear interpolation is adequate to obtain abridged life tables for other calendar years, it is inadequate to graduate these abridged life tables to single years of age. Nonlinear interpolation procedures must be used instead. Interpolation of the ℓ_x values in each abridged life table to single years of age is accomplished by means of a regression approach (Coale and Demeny 1966:20–23) for ages 1–4 and a matrix approach to polynomial interpolation (Feeney 1974) for subsequent five-year age groups. The end result is a set of ℓ_x values by single years of age for each intermediate calendar year. Single-year values of L_x (person-years of exposure) for ages 1–84 are obtained from the single-year values of ℓ_x using the formula $L_x = .5(\ell_x + \ell_{x+1})$. The interpolation of abridged ℓ_x values to single years of age is described in more detail in Appendix A (see also Retherford 1978). A computer subprogram is available for carrying out the various interpolations.

Estimation of infant and child mortality. When life tables for years near the census are not available, the Brass method of estimating infant and child mortality (Brass 1975) or Feeney's extension of Brass's method (Feeney 1980) can be applied to census data on number of children ever born and number of children still living. From these data Brass's method provides estimates of child mortality levels prevailing before the census, and Feeney's extension of Brass's method provides estimates of both child mortality levels and trends. Brass's and Feeney's methods are convenient because they can be used to estimate child mortality from the same data set from which the own-children fertility estimates are derived.

Brass's and Feeney's methods of estimating infant and child mortality require the same data on proportions of surviving children among all children ever born to women of ages 15 to 64, classified by woman's age in five-year age groups. The infant and child mortality estimates generated from these data can be matched to model life tables such as one of the model life tables developed by Coale and Demeny (1966, 1983) or Brass (1975). In this way complete life tables spanning all ages are obtained. A computer subprogram is available for computing the infant and child mortality estimates and matching them to complete life tables.

Sampling variability of own-children fertility estimates. A rough estimate of the standard error of $_5F_a(t - x - 1)$, denoted below simply as F, is

$$s_F = k\{[(1 - f)F(1 - F)]/(\tilde{W} - 1)\}^{.5}, \tag{2.14}$$

where $k = r_{0 \leftarrow x}/_5R^f_{a \leftarrow a+x+.5}$, f is the sampling function, and $\tilde{W} = {}_5W_a \, {}_5U^w_a$. A rough estimate of the standard error of the TFR is

$$s_{TFR} = 5(\Sigma_i s^2_{F_i})^{.5}. \tag{2.15}$$

A more extended discussion of sampling variability, including derivations of the above formulae, is contained in Appendix B.

Data collection requirements

One of the great advantages of the own-children method is that it can be applied to existing censuses and household surveys, so that no new data collection is required. If an application of the own-children method is anticipated, however, it is desirable to design the census or survey to facilitate the application. Each respondent should be identified with a household identifier, so that persons within the same household can be treated as a block. (This is necessary for matching children to mothers within the same household.) Age, sex, and marital status are basic questions that should always be asked. Age should be coded in single years.

Questions on number of children ever born and number of children still living facilitate both the matching of children to mothers and the derivation of mortality estimates. Matching may be further facilitated and made more accurate by coding the line number (or person number, as it is sometimes called) or mother (if present) in the household listing, for each person below the age of 15 (or 20) in the household. Alternatively, if matching is based primarily on relationship information, sufficiently detailed relationship codes should be used to enable an accurate match in almost all cases. If, for example, adoption is prevalent in the population, then one of the relationship codes should be "adopted child of household head," since otherwise adopted children will be erroneously matched and treated as own children. Normally, if relationship to the head is to be ascertained anyway, an extra question on the mother's line number is not needed unless households are large and complex, with many ambiguous matches, as in certain Pacific island populations. A slight, further improvement in the estimates can be realized if it is ascertained whether the mother of each child under age 15 is alive or dead, but this improvement may not be large enough to justify an additional item in a questionnaire usually crowded with other, more essential items.

Two extensions of the basic own-children method involve estimation of age–duration-specific birth rates (with duration measured since first marriage) and age–parity-specific birth rates. A question on year of or age at first marriage is necessary to calculate age–duration-specific birth rates, and a question on number of children ever born (parity) is necessary to calculate age–parity-specific birth rates. A question on birth order of each child under age 15 is needed to calculate age–parity-specific birth rates for years further back than the first year before the census.

CHAPTER 3

Methodological Extensions

Marital birth rates for currently married women

Estimates of age-specific birth rates for currently married women are obtained in the following way: First, age-specific proportions currently married in five-year age groups are obtained from two or more censuses spanning the estimation period. These proportions are interpolated or extrapolated linearly, from two censuses at a time, to get age-specific proportions currently married in five-year age groups for other years during the estimation period.

More precisely, the procedure for interpolation or extrapolation is as follows: Let $P_a(t)$ denote the age-specific proportion currently married at ages a to $a + 5$ at time t. Let t_1 denote the date of the first census and t_2 denote the date of the second census. Then for any other time, t,

$$P_a(t) = P_a(t_1) + [(t - t_1)/(t_2 - t_1)][P_a(t_2) - P_a(t_1)]. \tag{3.1}$$

In this way one obtains a table, or array, of age-specific proportions currently married, with age in five-year age groups along one dimension and time in single calendar years (or midpoints of time periods) along the other dimension. The original own-children analysis yields a corresponding array of age-specific birth rates for all women regardless of marital status. Term-by-term division of the second array by the first array yields a third array of age-specific birth rates for currently married women. This procedure assumes that all births occur within marriage. In some populations this is a poor assumption, particularly at the younger reproductive ages.

Equation (3.1) is also used to interpolate or extrapolate age-specific proportions never married or single. From the age-specific proportions single, one can calculate the singulate mean age at marriage (SMAM) at the midpoints of calendar years or groups of calendar years (Hajnal 1953). SMAM is used as a summary index of nuptiality. If a question on age at first marriage is included in the census, mean age at first marriage (MAM) can be calculated directly, and the use of SMAM is unnecessary.

The m *index of marital fertility control.* From the own-children estimates of age-specific birth rates for currently married women, one can compute the Coale–Trussell m index of marital fertility control (Coale and Trussell 1974, 1975, 1978). This index measures the deviation of the observed age pattern of marital fertility from the typical age pattern of natural marital fertility, where it is assumed that the deviation of observed fertility from natural fertility results from deliberate family limitation. Natural marital fertility is defined as marital fertility in the absence of deliberate family limitation.

The m index depends on the shape of the age-specific marital fertility schedule, not on the level of marital fertility. In the natural fertility situation, the shape of the schedule is convex-upward throughout the reproductive age range, whereas in the family limitation situation it is concave-upward at the upper end of the range. For purposes of constructing the m index, the standard age schedule of natural marital fertility is obtained as the arithmetic average of ten of the schedules designated by Henry (1961). If the observed age-specific marital fertility schedule has the same shape as that of the standard age-specific natural marital fertility schedule, $m = 0$. If the shape of the observed schedule deviates from the shape of the standard schedule by an amount that is the average deviation of 43 reasonably reliable marital fertility schedules in the early 1960s, representing a range of differences in the extent of fertility control, then $m = 1$. Values of m higher than 1 are also possible.

Not only an overall m, but also age-specific m's can be computed. If the model age-specific marital fertility schedule on which the m index is based fits the observed schedule perfectly, the overall m and the age-specific m's all have the same value. Thus the variance of the age-specific m's provides an indication of the validity of the m index. In applications where the age-specific m's are not consistent, age misreporting is frequently a contributing cause of the inconsistency.

The m index of marital fertility control is useful in instances where direct measures of the extent of contraceptive use for family limitation purposes is unavailable. These instances occur mostly for detailed cross-classified socioeconomic categories and small geographic areas, for which contraceptive use rates are usually unavailable but for which census samples provide sufficient numbers of cases for computation of own-children fertility estimates.

A computer program developed by the Office of Population Research at Princeton University is used to compute the *m* index and related statistics.

Illustrative results for Sri Lanka. Table 3.1 and Figure 3.1 provide illustrative results for Sri Lanka, again based on application of the own-children method to the 1981 Census. Table 3.1 shows values of TFRs, marital total fertility rates (MTFRs), *m,* and SMAM by education and rural–urban residence, aggregated over five-year time periods. MTFRs are calculated by adding age-specific birth rates for currently married women and dividing the sum by five. The MTFRs in the table exclude marital fertility at ages 15–19, which is high but based on very few married women, since Sri Lankan women tend to marry late. The results are aggregated over five-year time periods to suppress unnecessary detail and to smooth annual fluctuations. Annual fluctuations are especially large for the *m* index, which is highly sensitive to age misreporting—much more so than the own-children estimates of marital fertility themselves, on which the *m* index is based.

Table 3.1. Total fertility rates, marital total fertility rates, singulate mean ages at marriage, and values of the *m* index of marital fertility control, by completed years of education and urban–rural residence, derived by applying the own-children method of fertility estimation to the 1981 Census: Sri Lanka, 1966–70 to 1976–80

Education and measure	Total			Urban			Rural		
	1966 –70	1971 –75	1976 –80	1966 –70	1971 –75	1976 –80	1966 –70	1971 –75	1976 –80
0–5									
TFR	5,328	4,487	4,215	5,355	4,118	3,644	5,285	4,529	4,291
MTFR	5,992	5,218	5,115	5,986	4,828	4,628	5,944	5,257	5,170
SMAM	21.4	21.7	22.1	21.2	21.8	22.4	21.5	21.8	22.0
m	.56	.56	.74	.70	.79	.83	.54	.64	.73
6–10									
TFR	4,269	3,538	3,146	4,306	3,227	2,632	4,332	3,697	3,358
MTFR	6,612	5,466	4,870	6,688	5,148	4,255	6,682	5,639	5,113
SMAM	25.0	25.1	25.1	24.8	25.2	25.5	25.1	25.1	25.0
m	.75	.80	.86	.83	.95	.97	.71	.74	.81
11+									
TFR	3,097	2,556	2,038	3,219	2,424	1,762	3,140	2,716	2,256
MTFR	6,521	5,567	4,604	6,638	5,252	3,954	6,816	5,946	5,120
SMAM	27.6	28.3	28.9	26.6	27.4	28.3	28.3	28.8	29.3
m	.69	.63	.76	.78	.72	.90	.66	.58	.68

Source: Ratnayake, Retherford, and Sivasubramaniam (1984:26).

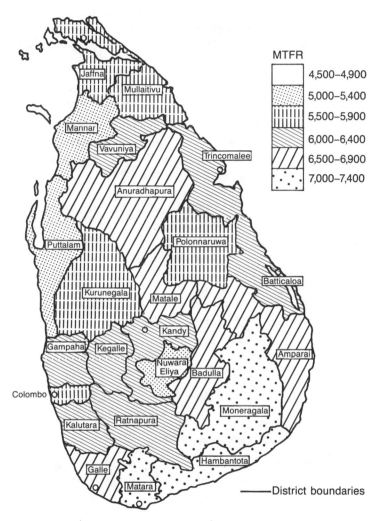

Figure 3.1. Own-children estimates of marital total fertility rates, by district, derived from the 1981 Census: Sri Lanka, 1966–70

Source: Ratnayake, Retherford, and Sivasubramaniam (1984:46).

Whereas Table 3.1 illustrates socioeconomic detail, Figure 3.1 illustrates geographic detail, summarized conveniently by means of a map. The map shows the level of the marital total fertility rate for the twenty-four districts of Sri Lanka for the time period 1966–70. Similar maps have been constructed for the periods 1971–75 and 1976–80, and for the TFR, SMAM, and m (Ratnayake, Retherford, and Sivasubramaniam 1984).

Ever-marital birth rates by duration since first marriage

When a question on age at first marriage is asked in a census, the own-children method may be extended to estimate birth rates by duration since first marriage for ever-married women. Of course, one cannot simply substitute the duration variable for the age variable, because reverse-survival factors are by nature age-specific, not duration-specific. An intermediate step must consist of estimating birth rates specific for both age and duration, which may then be aggregated over age to provide purely duration-specific measures. This extension of the method yields estimates of age–duration-specific ever-marital birth rates, age-specific ever-marital birth rates, duration-specific ever-marital birth rates, and two measures of ever-marital total fertility, one obtained by summing age-specific ever-marital birth rates over age and the other by summing duration-specific ever-marital birth rates over duration.

As in the case of the original method, the logic of this extension of the method is most easily explained with continuous functions. Accordingly, we again present both a continuous formulation and a discrete formulation.

Continuous formulation. We have the following definitions:

$f_{a,d}(t)$: Instantaneous age–duration-specific birth rate for ever-married women of age a and duration d at time t

$C_{x,a,d}$: Number of own children aged x of mothers of age a and duration d enumerated in the census

$B_{a,d}(t)$: Number of births to women of age a and duration d at time t

$W_{a,d}(t)$: Number of women of age a and duration d at time t

where duration since first marriage is determined as the difference between age at the time of the census and age at first marriage. Other quantities are defined as in the continuous formulation of the original method in the previous chapter. Again for simplicity, we consider that numbers of women and children at the time of the census have already been adjusted for underenumeration, age misreporting, and non-own children, and that mortality has been constant over the estimation period. Then, with t denoting the time of the census,

$$B_{a-x,d-x}(t - x) = C_{x,a,d}(\ell_0/_x) \tag{3.1}$$

$$W_{a-x,d-x}(t - x) = W_{a,d}(t)\,(\ell^f_{a-x}/\ell^f_a) \tag{3.2}$$

$$f_{a-x,d-x}(t - x) = B_{a-x,d-x}(t - x)/W_{a-x,d-x}(t - x). \tag{3.3}$$

Note that the age and duration associated with an own-children estimate of an age–duration-specific birth rate are the age and duration obtaining at the time of childbirth, not the time of the census. When these age–duration-specific rates are tabulated by characteristics such as education, however, these latter characteristics normally pertain to the time of the census.

Discrete formulation. We have the following definitions, in addition to the earlier definitions for the discrete formulation of the original method:

$F_{a,d}(t)$: Single-year central age–duration-specific ever-marital birth rate for women of age a to $a + 1$ and duration d to $d + 1$ during the calendar year t to $t + 1$

$C_{x,a,d}$: Number of own children aged x to $x + 1$ of mothers of age a to $a + 1$ and duration d to $d + 1$ enumerated in the census

$B_{a,d}(t)$: Births during the period t to $t + 1$ to women of duration d to $d + 1$ who were aged a to $a + 1$ at time t

$W_{a,d}(t)$: Ever-married women of age a to $a + 1$ and duration d to $d + 1$ at time t.

Other quantities are defined as in the discrete formulation of the original method in the previous chapter.

Again duration, d, is determined as the difference between age at the time of the census and age at first marriage. But the census normally provides these latter ages only in completed years, not as exact ages. This imprecision is handled in the following way: Denote age at first marriage in completed years by A_m. Denote age in completed years at the time of the census by a. Consider women at the time of the census for whom $a - A_m = 0$. For these women d ranges from exactly 0 to exactly 1. Hence we assign them to $W_{a,0}$. Suppose $a - A_m = 1$. For these women d ranges from exactly 0 to exactly 2. Hence we assign half of them to $W_{a,0}$ and the other half to $W_{a,1}$. Suppose $a - A_m = 2$. For these women d ranges from exactly 1 to exactly 3. Hence we assign half of them to $W_{a,1}$ and the other half to $W_{a,2}$. The procedure is similar for higher values of $a - A_m$. Parallel assignments are made for the children, $C_{x,a,d}$, of these women. Children for whom $x > a - A_m$ are considered illegitimate and are omitted from consideration. In this way values of $W_{a,d}$ and $C_{x,a,d}$ at the time of the census are obtained.

In the formulas for the discrete case, variable mortality and adjustments for underenumeration and age misreporting and for non-own children are taken explicitly into account. For census enumeration at time t we have

$$B_{a,d}(t - x - 1) = .5[C_{x,a+x+1,d+x} + C_{x,a+x+1,d+x+1}] \, U^c_{x,a+x+1} \, V_x \, r_{0 \leftarrow x}$$
$$\text{for } d > 0 \tag{3.4}$$

$$B_{a,0}(t - x - 1) = [C_{x,a+x+1,x} + .5 \, C_{x,a+x+1,x+1}] \, U^c_{x,a+x+1} \, V_x \, r_{0 \leftarrow x}$$
$$\text{for } d = 0 \tag{3.5}$$

$$W_{a,d}(t - x - 1) = W_{a+x+1,d+x+1}(t) \, U^w_{a+x+1} \, R^f_{a \leftarrow a+x+1} \tag{3.6}$$

$$F_{a,d}(t - x - 1) = [B_{a-1,d}(t - x - 1) + B_{a,d}(t + x + 1)]/$$
$$[W_{a,d}(t - x - 1) + W_{a,d}(t - x)]. \tag{3.7}$$

To clarify equation (3.4), consider, for example, the case of $x = 0$. We view $C_{0,a+1,d}$ as concentrated at $d + 0.5$ and $C_{0,a+1,d+1}$ as concentrated at $d + 1.5$. We then view the average of these two quantities as concentrated at exactly $d + 1$. Therefore, one year ago the average marriage duration of mothers of these children was exactly d. Thus the births over the past year, $B_{a,d}(t - 1)$, corresponding to these children, occurred on average between exact durations d and $d + 1$, which is what we desire. Similar reasoning applies to the case of nonzero x.

A special case, given in equation (3.5), occurs when $d = 0$. Were equation (3.4) to be used, half the children, $C_{x,a+x+1,x}$ in equation (3.5), would end up assigned to $B_{a,-1}(t - x - 1)$, in the category of illegitimate births. Since this is inadmissable, given our earlier assumptions, equation (3.5) simply constrains all these births to $B_{a,0}(t - x - 1)$. Note, however, that not all births are being constrained to positive durations. Births corresponding to children for whom $x > a - A_m$ do not appear at all in equations (3.4) and (3.5). These births are considered illegitimate and are ignored.

In equation (3.6) the numerator and denominator are again each obtained by an averaging procedure. As before, multiplicative factors of 0.5 cancel in the quotient and are not shown.

Note that because a good deal of averaging is incorporated into the procedure, the rates by single years of duration are substantially smoothed. This smoothing does not pose a problem at higher durations, but it may introduce some distortions at very short durations of one or two years.

From equation (3.7) it is evident that numerators and denominators of rates are computed separately. They are stored in a three-dimensional birth array and a three-dimensional woman array, the dimensions of which are woman's age, woman's marriage duration, and calendar year, each specified by single years of age or time. The two arrays may be collapsed or grouped along any dimension before they are divided term by term to get the corresponding array of rates. For example, if the arrays are completely collapsed along the age dimension, dividing the birth array by the woman array yields an array of birth rates specified by duration only for each calendar year. Thus the method yields age-specific ever-marital birth rates and duration-specific ever-marital birth rates as well as age–duration-specific ever-marital birth rates. Normally ages are grouped into standard five-year age intervals.

Age-specific ever-marital birth rates in five-year age groups may be summed and the sum multiplied by five to yield a measure of the ever-marital total fertility rate, denoted EMTFR$_a$, where subscript a denotes summation over age. In late-marrying populations, EMTFR$_a$ summed over ages 15–49 is not a very good fertility measure because it assigns the same weight to the birth rate at ages 15–19, which is high but based on very few ever-married women and births, as it assigns to birth rates in other age groups. Since fertility trends and differentials at ages 15–19 often differ substantially from trends and differentials at other ages, a measure that accords undue weight to fertility at ages 15–19 can produce a distorted view of overall fertility trends and differentials. Moreover, the own-children estimates of fertility at ages 15–19 are less reliable than at higher ages. This difficulty may be avoided by summing rates over ages 20–49 instead of 15–49.

Duration-specific birth rates can be summed to yield an alternative measure, EMTFR$_d$, where subscript d denotes summation over duration. The weighting problem then disappears, because there are many ever-married women and births at duration 0. Therefore, none of the durations need be omitted from the summation.

In applying the above procedure, the same age-specific reverse-survival ratios are used regardless of duration, because age-specific death rates are almost never available by duration since first marriage. The error introduced by not specifying mortality by duration as well as by age is very small. The impact of mortality estimation errors on the own-children fertility estimates is discussed in more detail in Chapter 4.

Figure 3.2 shows trends in EMTFR$_d$, derived by applying the own-children method to the 1980 Census of the Republic of Korea. Separate

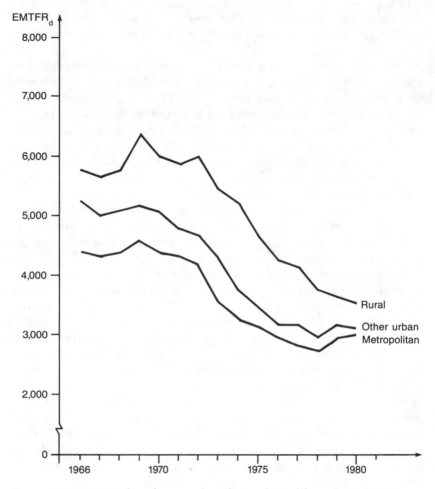

Figure 3.2. EMTFR$_d$, by urban–rural residence, derived from the 1980 Census: Republic of Korea, 1966–80

Source: Retherford, Cho, and Kim (1984:556).

trends are shown for three categories of urban–rural residence. This application involved an instructive analysis of estimation errors, discussed in detail in Chapter 4.

Age–parity-specific birth rates and birth probabilities

Censuses typically include a question on woman's parity, or number of children she has ever borne. With this information the own-children method can be extended to estimate age–parity-specific birth rates and birth probabilities, but only for the year previous to the census. The birth probabilities can be aggregated to yield estimates of parity progression ratios. Two simplifying assumptions are that (1) age-specific mortality does not vary by birth order of child or parity of woman, and (2) no woman gives birth to more than one child per year. Neither of these assumptions introduces serious error.

Because parity is a discrete variable, continuous functions are inappropriate for explaining the methodology. Therefore, the explanation that follows is framed solely in discrete terms.

We have the following definitions:

$F_{a,i}(t)$: Single-year central age–parity-specific birth rate for women of age a and parity i during calendar year t to $t+1$

$g_{a,i}(t)$: Single-year gross age–parity-specific birth probability for calendar year t to $t+1$

$g_{a,i}^{*}(t)$: Single-year net age–parity-specific birth probability for calendar year t to $t+1$

$C_{x,a,i}$: Number of own children aged x to $x+1$ of mothers of age a to $a+1$ and parity i enumerated in the census

$B_{a,i}(t)$: Births during the calendar year t to $t+1$ to women of age a to $a+1$ and parity i at time t

$W_{a,i}(t)$: Number of women of age a to $a+1$ and parity i at time t

Other quantities are defined as in the discrete formulation of the original method in Chapter 2.

Let us first consider the calculation of central age–parity-specific birth rates for the year previous to the census. With t denoting the time of the census, we have that

$$B_{a,i}(t-1) = C_{0,a+1,i+1}\, U_{0,a}^{c}\, V_0\, r_{0 \leftarrow 0} \tag{3.8}$$

$$W_{a,i}(t-1) = W_{a+1,i}(t)\, U_{a+1}^{w}\, R_{a \leftarrow a+1}^{f}$$
$$- B_{a,i-1}(t-1) + B_{a,i}(t-1) \tag{3.9}$$

$$F_{a,i}(t-1) = [B_{a-1,i}(t-1) + B_{a,i}(t-1)]/$$
$$[W_{a,i}(t) + W_{a,i}(t-1)]. \tag{3.10}$$

The numerator and denominator of formula (3.10) are each obtained by an averaging procedure, and again factors of 0.5 in the numerator and denominator cancel in the quotient and are not shown. Figure 3.3 as well as Figure 2.1 in the previous chapter illustrate the logic of these formulas.

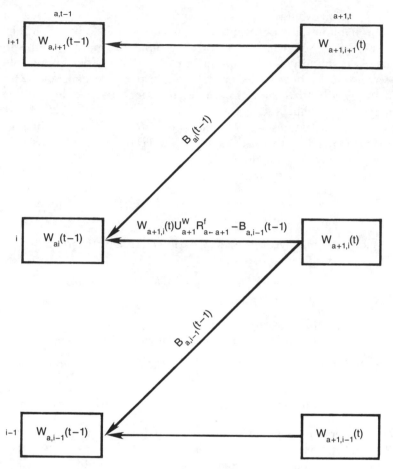

Figure 3.3. Age–parity reverse-survival diagram for calculating $W_{a,i}(t-1)$

Source: Retherford and Cho (1978:571).
Note: Expressions written above arrows denote numbers of reverse-survived women.

The last parity group in formulas (3.8) to (3.10) will be open-ended, say 7+. In this case $i-1$ is interpreted as parity 6, i as parity 7+, and $i+1$ as parity 8+; and the last term in formula (3.9), $B_{a,i}(t-1)$, is omitted. Otherwise, the calculation resembles that for the earlier single parities.

The computation of age–parity-specific birth probabilities assumes that at time t women aged $a-1$ to $a+1$ of parity i and their births are spread evenly over this age interval. These women are then viewed as concentrated at the midpoint of the interval, i.e. at exact age a. We have then for the net age–parity-specific birth probability

$$g_{a,i}^{*}(t - 1) = [B_{a,i}(t - 1) + B_{a-1,i}(t - 1)]/$$
$$[W_{a,i}(t - 1) + W_{a-1,i}(t - 1)]. \tag{3.11}$$

Again Figure 2.1 aids in understanding this formula. As before, the numerator and denominator are each obtained by an averaging process, and again factors of 0.5 in the numerator and denominator cancel in the quotient and are not shown.

The birth probability in equation (3.11) is "net" because it incorporates the effects of mortality. The numbers of women at risk are eroded to a greater or lesser extent, depending on the level of mortality, which affects the number of births over the interval but not the initial population at risk. The "gross" age–parity-specific birth probability, which would hold in the absence of mortality, is somewhat higher than the net probability and is easily calculated from the net probability and the life tables as follows:

For the net probability we have

$$B_{a,i}^{*}(t) = g_{a,i}^{*}(t) \ W_{a,i}^{*}(t) \tag{3.12}$$

where B^{*} and W^{*} denote numerator and denominator on the right-hand side of (3.11), each multiplied by 0.5 and with $t - 1$ replaced by t. We assume that deaths are spread evenly over the year and that instantaneous birth rates are constant over the year and are the same for those who die as for those who survive. Hence, on average, women who die have half as many births during the year as they would have had, had they survived. The proportion dying over the interval is q_a. We can therefore rewrite (3.12) as

$$B_{a,i}^{*}(t) = W_{a,i}^{*}(t) \ g_{a,i}(t) - .5 \ W_{a,i}^{*}(t) \ q_a \ g_{a,i}(t). \tag{3.13}$$

Equating the right-hand sides of (3.12) and (3.13) and solving for the gross birth probability, $g_{a,i}(t)$, we obtain

$$g_{a,i}(t) = g_{a,i}^{*}(t)/(1 - .5 \ q_a). \tag{3.14}$$

This formula allows conversion of $g_{a,i}^{*}(t)$ to $g_{a,i}(t)$ and vice versa.

Gross and net age–parity-specific birth probabilities can be used to construct gross and net fertility tables of the life table type. Such tables indicate numbers of "survivors" at each age and parity, starting with an initial cohort or radix of women of parity 0 at age 15.

The fertility table calculations, along the lines of those for an ordinary life table, are straightforward. Let $b_{a,i}$ denote fertility table births to women of parity i between exact ages a and $a + 1$, and let $\ell_{a,i}$ denote the number of women of parity i at exact age a. The fertility table starts at age 15 with $\ell_{15,0}$ set equal to, say, 100,000. In the "gross" fertility table, with mortality ignored, we have that

$$b_{a,i} = \ell_{a,i}\, g_{a,i} \tag{3.15}$$

$$\ell_{a+1,i} = \ell_{a,i} - b_{a,i} + b_{a,i-1}. \tag{3.16}$$

These formulas are applied to one age at a time, by varying parity systematically within each age before progressing to the next age. In this way the entire fertility table is generated. From the fertility table, period parity progression ratios between parities i and $i + 1$ may be calculated as

$$\text{PPR}_i = \Sigma_a\, b_{a,i+1} / \Sigma_a\, b_{a,i}. \tag{3.17}$$

Many other useful fertility measures can also be calculated from such fertility tables. If desired, net fertility tables that incorporate mortality may also be calculated. (Special procedures are necessary when parities are grouped beyond a certain point—say, single parities to 6 followed by 7+; see Retherford and Cho 1978.)

Table 3.2 shows gross age–parity-specific birth probabilities for the United States in 1969, derived by applying the own-children method to the 1970 Census. In Chapter 4 we analyze the accuracy of these estimates by comparing them with parallel estimates derived from vital registration.

Birth rates for men instead of women

As mentioned earlier, own-children estimates of age-specific birth rates and derived measures can be computed for men as well as for women, yielding births per thousand men at risk instead of births per thousand women at risk (Retherford and Sewell 1986). When this is done, the fertility estimates are readily tabulated by men's characteristics. This is of particular interest for such characteristics as occupation and income, since in most populations men tend to be the main income earners.

This modification of the own-children method is necessary if one wants fertility estimates by men's characteristics, because it is not possible to tabulate the own-children fertility estimates for women by husbands' characteristics. Women with husbands are by definition currently married, and application of the basic own-children method to currently married women does not yield satisfactory results. Results are less than satisfactory because one does not know whether a woman who was mar-

Table 3.2. Gross age–parity-specific birth probabilities derived from the 1970
Census: United States, 1969

Age	\multicolumn{9}{c}{Parity}

Age	0	1	2	3	4	5	6	7+
15	12	112	63	—[a]	—	—	—	—
16	21	116	81	97	—	—	—	—
17	40	155	118	158	41	—	—	—
18	66	200	172	170	122	228	—	—
19	91	212	189	192	205	201	269	—
20	109	216	191	221	210	134	409	—
21	123	236	205	231	175	185	329	49
22	132	254	189	198	179	243	162	59
23	139	259	166	179	200	211	149	62
24	140	256	154	173	187	171	193	138
25	136	258	149	156	162	174	146	154
26	132	249	142	140	152	143	126	106
27	129	231	131	125	141	121	217	95
28	115	213	122	109	118	126	210	126
29	96	185	120	91	96	119	140	112
30	85	164	108	83	84	105	130	92
31	65	144	86	74	72	78	94	105
32	48	120	70	57	65	55	72	106
33	47	91	59	53	60	54	95	87
34	42	77	52	51	54	51	89	93
35	35	71	49	45	45	50	78	97
36	26	50	41	38	37	49	73	90
37	22	38	30	31	34	39	58	94
38	17	35	23	23	28	36	53	88
39	11	26	16	16	21	26	42	78
40	8	17	14	11	14	18	27	69
41	5	12	8	8	13	16	23	51
42	5	9	4	8	11	14	21	35
43	5	6	4	6	9	12	15	34
44	5	3	3	4	5	6	11	26
45	3	3	2	2	2	2	9	17
46	1	3	2	1	4	3	3	12
47	1	3	1	2	2	5	4	4
48	2	2	1	1	0	2	3	3
49	2	2	1	1	0	1	1	4

Source: Retherford and Cho (1978:575).
[a]Blank cells denote probabilities based on denominators of fewer than ten women.

ried at the time of the census was married or unmarried at times prior to the census. Thus the estimated rates for years prior to the census pertain to an ambiguous mix of unmarried and married women.

This extension of the method to men requires modification of the matching algorithm, in order to match children to fathers instead of mothers. The results are less precise than those for women, for two major reasons. First, censuses do not normally ask men the number of children they have fathered and the number of those who are still living. Since these questions are used, when available, to improve the accuracy of the child–parent matching procedure, the absence of these questions for men increases the number of matching errors. Second, when spouses divorce or otherwise separate, the children generally accompany the mother rather than the father. The own-children methodology can match such children to a mother but not a father, or at least not to the correct father. Therefore, the volume of unmatched (non-own) children is larger in the male than in the female version of the own-children procedure. Because of less precise matching and larger numbers of non-own children that must be allocated, the own-children method produces fertility estimates that are less accurate for men than for women. But the estimates for men are still sufficiently accurate for many purposes.

The calculation formulas for computing fertility estimates for men are virtually the same as those presented earlier for computing fertility estimates for women. The two principal differences are that in the former case men are substituted for women in the equations and the reproductive age range is extended by five years, to age 55. Births beyond age 55 for men are ignored in the current version of the computer program, which has been applied to U.S. data for the state of Wisconsin to yield estimates of fertility for men who never completed high school (Retherford and Sewell 1986).

Decomposition of fertility change into components

When the own-children method is applied to large census samples, it provides fertility estimates by detailed characteristics. When these detailed fertility estimates are available from two or more censuses, they may be used to decompose the change in the total fertility rate into components (Retherford and Ogawa 1978; Retherford and Cho 1981). The method is explained by means of an example, as follows:

Consider a change in the TFR, where the TFR is calculated as $5 \sum_a F_a$, and where F_a is the age-specific birth rate for the five-year age group beginning at age a. Suppose we write F_a as a weighted sum of age–education-specific birth rates, where each weight $k_{a,e}$ is the proportion of the age group a to $a + 5$ with education e (e.g., none, primary, or more than primary). Then

$$\text{TFR} = 5 \, \Sigma_{a,e} \, k_{a,e} \, F_{a,e} \qquad\qquad (3.18)$$

and

$$\Delta\text{TFR} = 5 \, \Sigma_{a,e} \, \bar{F}_{a,e} \, \Delta k_{a,e} + 5 \, \Sigma_{a,e} \, \bar{k}_{a,e} \, \Delta F_{a,e} \qquad\qquad (3.19)$$

where the symbol Δ denotes change and where $\bar{F}_{a,e}$ and $\bar{k}_{a,e}$, pertaining to the a–eth age–education group, are average values over the period obtained by summing beginning and end values and dividing by two. We thus obtain a sum of two principal contributions to ΔTFR, the first of which can be interpreted as stemming from changes in population composition by education and the second from changes in age–education-specific birth rates. Each of these two principal contributions can be further classified by age if so desired.

The above decomposition method can be extended to more variables by decomposing $\Delta F_{a,e}$ in the same way as ΔTFR. Suppose we introduce variables in the order (after age) of education (e), residence (r), and marital status (m). Education consists of, say, three categories (none, some primary, more than primary), residence of two (urban and rural), and marital status of two (currently married and not currently married). We assume that all births occur within marriage. The final decomposition is then

$$\begin{aligned}
\Delta\text{TFR} = {} &5 \, \Sigma_{a,e} \, \bar{F}_{a,e} \, \Delta k_{a,e} + 5 \, \Sigma_{a,e,r} \, \bar{k}_{a,e} \, \bar{F}_{a,e,r} \, \Delta k_{a,e,r} \\
&+ 5 \, \Sigma_{a,e,r,m} \, \bar{k}_{a,e} \, \bar{k}_{a,e,r} \, \bar{F}_{a,e,r,m} \, \Delta k_{a,e,r,m} \\
&+ 5 \, \Sigma_{a,e,r,m} \, \bar{k}_{a,e} \, \bar{k}_{a,e,r} \, \bar{k}_{a,e,r,m} \, \Delta F_{a,e,r,m},
\end{aligned} \qquad (3.20)$$

with symbols defined as follows:

$k_{a,e}$: Proportion of the ath age group (a to $a + 5$) with education e (females only)

$k_{a,e,r}$: Proportion of the a–eth age–education group with residence r

$k_{a,e,r,m}$: Proportion of the a–e–rth age–education–residence group with marital status m

$F_{a,e,r,m}$: Age–education–residence–marital-status-specific birth rate.

The various k-values can be tabulated directly from the census. Birth rates for all women, regardless of marital status, can be tabulated by education and residence using the original version of the own-children method outlined in the previous chapter. Birth rates by education and

Table 3.3. Percentage decomposition of changes in the total fertility rate due to changes in residence, education, marital status, and fertility: Republic of Korea, 1960–75

Period and age group	Residence	Education	Marital status	Fertility	Total
1960–66					
15–29	7.0	8.1	−5.3	15.6	25.3
30–49	6.3	6.9	−1.8	63.3	74.7
Total	13.3	15.0	−7.2	78.9	100.0
					(−1,381)
1966–70					
15–29	24.5	16.5	−6.9	−21.4	12.8
30–49	17.2	19.7	−14.0	64.2	87.1
Total	41.7	36.2	−20.7	42.9	100.0
					(−338)
1970–75					
15–29	2.6	4.2	18.9	1.7	27.3
30–49	4.6	3.4	−0.7	65.4	72.6
Total	7.1	7.6	18.1	67.2	100.0
					(−1,052)
1966–75					
15–29	9.7	8.1	11.4	−5.2	23.9
30–49	8.4	7.7	−3.3	63.2	76.3
Total	18.2	15.8	8.0	58.0	100.0
					(−1,390)
1960–75					
15–29	6.9	6.7	4.4	6.6	24.6
30–49	5.8	6.5	−3.3	66.2	75.4
Total	12.8	13.2	1.2	72.8	100.0
					(−2,770)

Source: Retherford and Cho (1981:8).
Note: The change in the total fertility rate, per thousand women, is given in parentheses at the lower right of each panel.

residence for currently married women are then obtained using the methodology explained in the first section of this chapter.

The first of the five principal terms on the right side of equation (3.20) denotes the contribution to change in the TFR from changes in education composition. The second term denotes the contribution from changes in residence composition within education groups. The third term denotes the contribution from changes in marital status composition within education–residence groups. The fourth term denotes the contribution from changes in age–education–residence–marital-status-specific birth rates. Note that the size of the education contribution in equation (3.19) is unaffected by the addition of more compositional variables in equation (3.20), since terms beyond the first in equation (3.20) simply decompose further the fertility contribution in equation (3.19).

The order in which variables are introduced into the decomposition in equation (3.20) influences the results. In equation (3.20) education is introduced before residence. When residence is introduced before education, the residence contribution increases and the education contribution diminishes in size. Education might be introduced first if it is considered the most fundamental variable affecting the change. Or residence might be introduced first because the order of residence, education, and marital status reflects for most people a logical time sequence of life-cycle events. As is frequently true in stepwise multivariate techniques, there is some ambiguity and latitude of choice regarding the proper order of introduction of variables.

Table 3.3 provides illustrative results for the Republic of Korea, based on application of the own-children method to the censuses of 1960, 1966, 1970, and 1975 (Retherford and Cho 1981). In this example, residence was introduced before education. The necessary measures of population composition, k_x, $k_{x,r}$, $k_{x,r,e}$, $k_{x,r,e,m}$, were estimated for each census date and used to approximate population composition six months before the census, at the middle of the year for which fertility was estimated. The measures could have been interpolated back six months, but this degree of precision was deemed unnecessary. Values of $F_{x,r,e,m}$ were computed for the year previous to each census by applying the own-children method to each census.

CHAPTER 4

Evaluation and Analysis of Errors

The effect of matching errors on own-children fertility estimates

A common but usually unimportant source of bias in own-children estimates of fertility arises from matching errors, of which there are three major types: (1) mismatch, (2) misallocation of unmatched children, and (3) failure to record the existence of some children because they are living in a geographic area other than the study area in which the mother lives.

Mismatch error may occur from overmatching, whereby more children are matched to a woman than actually are hers biologically. A frequent source of overmatching is insufficient precision in the codes for relation to head of household, which are used in the computer algorithm for matching children to mothers. This algorithm checks for configurations of codes that constitute an admissable match. For example, if, for a given household, an adult male is reported as the head of household and there is a woman reported as wife of head and a child reported as child of head, the algorithm will respond to that particular configuration of codes by matching the child to the wife.

An example of insufficiently precise relationship codes is provided by the 1974 Census of American Samoa, in which the relationship codes were as follows:

1. head
2. wife of head
3. son, daughter, nephew, or niece of head
4. grandchild of head
5. brother, sister, brother-in-law, or sister-in-law of head
6. father, mother, father-in-law, or mother-in-law of head
7. other relative

8. no relation
9. unknown

With this set of relationship codes, various kinds of matching errors can arise. For example, because sons and daughters cannot be distinguished from nephews and nieces, it is possible to match erroneously a woman's niece or nephew to her.

Another instance of mismatch concerns adoption. Relationship codes in the censuses of the United States, for example, do not distinguish biological children from adopted children. Therefore, adopted children tend to be matched erroneously to adoptive mothers instead of being treated as non-own (unmatched) and allocated by means of the non-own adjustment factor.

The matching algorithm makes use of questions on age, marital status, and number of children ever born or still living, in addition to the question on relation to household head. The algorithm will not match children to mothers who are out of range on age. That is, the difference between a mother's age and a child's age must fall within the 15–50 range. The algorithm also will not match children to women who have never married, although this requirement can be relaxed if consensual unions are prevalent. And the algorithm will not match more children to a woman than the number she says are still living (or were ever born, if the question on number still living was not asked). The algorithm then attempts to match children to mothers, starting at the top of the household listing and working down. As many children as possible are matched to the first eligible mother before the algorithm proceeds to the next. Although age and marital status are always asked on censuses, number of children ever born and number of children still living are not always asked. In such cases the probability of overmatching is increased.

Mismatch may stem also from undermatching. This can occur when a relationship is wrongly reported or, less commonly, miscoded. In either case, a child may not be matched to its biological mother even when both are in the same household. This can happen, for example, if the household head refers affectionately to a child as a grandchild when in reality the relation is less direct. Undermatching can occur also as a consequence of underreporting of children ever born or children surviving; this form of undermatching is thought to be uncommon, however, since omitted children tend to be either dead or living elsewhere. As will be seen shortly, tests of alternative matching procedures suggest that undermatching is more common than overmatching, contrary to expectations.

If mismatch is statistically independent of mother's age, it will not distort the own-children estimates of age-specific birth rates because the children in question are taken into account one way or the other; i.e., they are either matched and included as own children, or they are classified as non-own and allocated. We shall see shortly, however, that mismatch occurs more frequently at some ages than at others, with the result that the age pattern of fertility is systematically distorted. But the overall level of fertility, as measured by the total fertility rate, tends to be affected very little.

The second type of matching error involves misallocation of unmatched, or non-own, children. If, for example, younger women are more likely than older women to be separated temporarily from their young children (owing, say, to labor migration of young women who leave children temporarily in the care of relatives), the distribution of non-own children of a given age by age of mother will be more concentrated at younger ages of mothers than is true of the distribution of own children of the same age by age of mother. In applying the own-children method in this situation, we do not know the ages of the mothers of the non-own children. We simply assume that non-own children of a given age are distributed by age of mother in the same way as own children of the same age. But this assumption introduces bias, because the non-own adjustment factor then effectively reallocates a certain proportion of non-own children from younger mothers to older mothers. As a consequence, the estimated age pattern of fertility is too low at the younger reproductive ages and too high at the older reproductive ages.

Misallocation of non-own children can occur not only across ages but also across other characteristics. For example, the distribution of non-own children of a given age by education of mother may be more concentrated at lower levels of education, where mortality and the risk of orphanhood are higher, than is true of the distribution of own children of the same age by education of mother. Non-own adjustment factors can be tabulated no more by education of mother than by age of mother, since the mothers of non-own children are unidentified. Thus the non-own adjustment is the same, regardless of education of mother. Fertility estimates by education are biased if the true adjustments for non-own children (as opposed to the estimated adjustments) differ by education of mother. Misallocation of non-own children has little impact on the fertility estimates if the non-own adjustment factors are small. But these factors are occasionally as high as 1.3 or 1.4 for older children. Then the potential for bias is greater.

The third type of matching error involves failure to record the existence of some children because they are living in a geographic area other than the study area in which the mother lives. In the case of large-scale in-migration to the study area, for example, women may leave children temporarily in the care of relatives at the point of origin until they become resettled at the destination. In this situation the own-children estimates of fertility in the destination area are downwardly biased. Bias from this source is probably very small, because migrants who are separated from their young children usually constitute a very small proportion of the population.

Illustrative analysis of the effect of mismatch on own-children fertility estimates for American Samoa and Indonesia. Not all of the matching errors discussed above have been studied empirically to assess directly the magnitude of their impact on own-children estimates of fertility. Mismatch errors have received the most attention, and they have been investigated for American Samoa with data from the 1974 Census, and for East Java with data from the 1976 Indonesian Intercensal Population Survey, also known as SUPAS II (Levin and Retherford 1982).

The American Samoan analysis was based on a virtually complete population count of 29,100 individuals, and the East Java analysis on a sample of 35,822 individuals. In each case the census included a special census question on mother's person number or line number in the household listing, completed for each child whose biological mother was in the same household. It was anticipated that the direct match based on mother's person number (MPN matching) would match fewer children than the indirect match based on relation to head of household (RHH matching), since there is, in the former case, less ambiguity about the mother–child relationship and therefore a reduced probability of erroneously matching the child when the biological mother is actually absent. The data allowed a test of this hypothesis, as well as an assessment of the effect of erroneous matches on the own-children estimates of fertility.

Although the American Samoa and East Java data sets are similar in that both allow MPN matching, they differ in some other respects. In American Samoa, adoption is common, households are generally large and complex, and the frequency of in- and out-migration (mainly to the United States) is very high, leading to frequent temporary separations of family members. Under these conditions the likelihood of mismatch was expected to be considerably higher for RHH matching than for MPN matching. In East Java, on the other hand, households are simpler and smaller and the population is less migratory; under these conditions the likelihood of mismatch was expected to be low for both types of matching.

The relationship codes in Indonesia are also more elaborate than in American Samoa, allowing more precise RHH matching. The relationship codes for American Samoa were given earlier (pages 36–37). The codes for Indonesia are as follows:

1. head
2. wife of head
3. own child of head
4. non-own child of head (adopted child or stepchild)
5. grandchild of head
6. parent of head
7. parent of wife of head
8. daughter-in-law or son-in-law of head
9. other family
10. other nonfamily
11. unknown

Because of more complex households, more frequent temporary family separations, and less precise relationship codes in American Samoa than in Indonesia, one expects MPN matching to improve the accuracy of the fertility estimates more for American Samoa than for East Java.

Table 4.1 shows the percentage that non-own children constitute of all children in each single-year age group according to type of match. As

Table 4.1. Non-own children as a percentage of all children, by type of matching: American Samoa, 1974, and East Java, 1976

Age	American Samoa, 1974		East Java, 1976	
	RHH	*MPN*	*RHH*	*MPN*
0	24.8	13.2	2.1	1.2
1	23.2	15.5	3.8	1.5
2	26.2	18.6	4.2	3.1
3	22.4	17.2	6.7	5.2
4	24.6	19.2	6.2	4.4
5	25.0	21.0	6.0	4.5
6	22.2	17.5	7.9	6.5
7	24.1	20.3	9.2	7.1
8	23.5	20.1	10.9	9.0
9	22.8	20.2	8.7	6.5
10	24.5	21.9	12.5	9.5
11	27.0	24.1	13.3	9.3
12	22.4	21.5	15.4	12.6
13	29.0	27.9	15.4	12.4
14	29.5	27.7	17.5	15.6

Source: Levin and Retherford (1982:12).
RHH—relation to head of household.
MPN—mother's person number.

expected, the percentage not matched is higher in American Samoa than in East Java. Also expected is the greater divergence between RHH and MPN matching in American Samoa than in East Java. The percentage not matched tends to rise steeply with age of child, mainly because older children are more likely than younger children to live in a household other than their mother's. An unanticipated exception is RHH matching in American Samoa. In this case the percentage not matched is unusually high among younger children, and the typical rise with age in the percentage not matched is largely eliminated. The difference between RHH and MPN matching in American Samoa is especially great for younger children.

The most startling finding in Table 4.1 is that in both American Samoa and Indonesia the percentage not matched is higher for RHH matching than for MPN matching, the reverse of what was anticipated. Further investigation of the American Samoan case showed that the MPN match produced 815 unmatched, or non-own, children. Of these only eleven were erroneously matched by the RHH match, indicating that over-matching by the RHH algorithm is not a serious problem. Offsetting these eleven children who were overmatched were 107 children who were correctly matched by MPN matching but not matched by RHH matching, owing to errors in relationship codes. These errors appear to consist mainly of respondent errors, not interviewer errors. Quite commonly, for example, the household head incorrectly reported a child as grandchild, while correctly reporting the child's mother (identified by MPN matching) as an "other relative" instead of a daughter or daughter-in-law as would be necessary if the child were truly a grandchild. If the household lacked an eligible daughter or daughter-in-law, RHH matching then incorrectly designated the child as non-own. This kind of error was especially common for very young children, for whom the reported grandparent–grandchild relationship evidently often reflects an affectionate social tie rather than a biological tie.

The results in Table 4.1 suggest that fertility estimates based alternatively on RHH and MPN matching should coincide approximately for East Java but diverge slightly for American Samoa, particularly in the years just previous to enumeration, for which fertility estimates are based on reverse survival of very young children. Figures 4.1 and 4.2 confirm this expectation. In the case of East Java, fertility estimates based alternatively on RHH and MPN matching differ by less than 2 percent, and usually less than 1 percent, over single calendar years between 1962 and 1976. In American Samoa, on the other hand, the discrepancy, though small in years close to 1960, increases for years closer to the census, reaching almost 4 percent in 1974. In American Samoa, estimates of

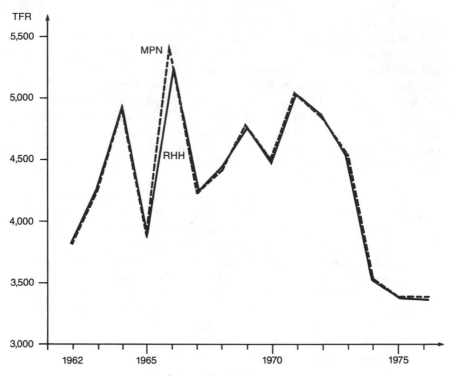

Figure 4.1. Own-children estimates of total fertility rates derived from the 1976 Indonesian Intercensal Population Survey, based alternatively on relationship to household head (RHH) and mother's person number (MPN): East Java, 1962–76

Source: Levin and Retherford (1982:12).

the total fertility rate based on RHH matching are consistently higher than estimates based on MPN matching. In East Java the much smaller discrepancies are in both directions and show no clear pattern. The consistent direction of the discrepancy in American Samoa stems from a systematic distortion in the age pattern of fertility, to which we now turn.

Table 4.2 examines the effects of alternative matching procedures on the age pattern of fertility. Calendar years are grouped into two five-year periods to minimize effects of heaping of children's ages on preferred digits on the fertility estimates. In East Java the difference between the age patterns of fertility estimated alternatively using RHH and MPN matching is inconsequential, consistent with the small differences in matching results and TFR estimates in Table 4.1 and Figure 4.1. In

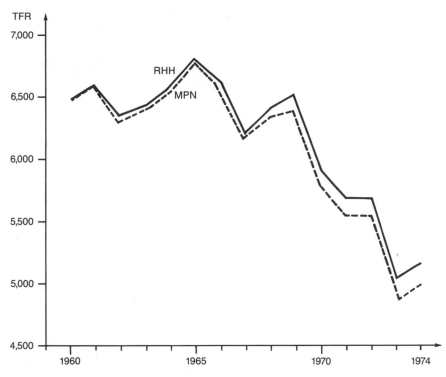

Figure 4.2. Own-children estimates of total fertility rates derived from the 1974 Census, based alternatively on relationship to household head (RHH) and mother's person number (MPN): American Samoa, 1960–74

Source: Levin and Retherford (1982:12).

American Samoa, however, RHH matching results in underestimates of fertility at the younger reproductive ages and overestimates at the older reproductive ages, especially for the second five-year period, 1968–72. This evidently occurs because RHH matching erroneously allocates too many children to older women and not enough to younger women, relative to results based on MPN matching. The likely underlying reasons for this misallocation have already been discussed.

Because the number of women in each five-year age group decreases with age, the shift of children from younger women to older women increases birth rates at the older reproductive ages more than it decreases birth rates at the younger reproductive ages. This effect probably explains why the TFR computed from age-specific birth rates based on

Table 4.2. Own-children estimates of age-specific birth rates and total fertility rates, by type of matching: American Samoa, 1963–72, and East Java, 1965–74

Country, period, and type of matching	Age group							
	15–19	*20–24*	*25–29*	*30–34*	*35–39*	*40–44*	*45–49*	*TFR*
American Samoa								
1963–67								
RHH	43	233	321	312	241	123	29	6,519
MPN	47	242	320	311	232	117	25	6,470
RHH/MPN	.923	.964	1.003	1.005	1.037	1.053	1.178	1.007
1968–72								
RHH	43	222	287	270	230	110	39	6,000
MPN	47	239	293	260	215	98	27	5,995
RHH/MPN	.925	.927	.979	1.037	1.067	1.126	1.435	1.001
East Java								
1965–69								
RHH	135	226	206	168	108	48	14	4,532
MPN	134	225	205	167	107	48	15	4,511
RHH/MPN	1.007	1.005	1.005	1.010	1.004	.996	.953	1.005
1970–74								
RHH	124	230	207	162	100	51	14	4,435
MPN	125	231	206	162	101	51	15	4,448
RHH/MPN	.989	.995	1.003	1.004	.997	1.007	.925	.997

Source: Levin and Retherford (1982:13).

RHH matching slightly but consistently exceeds the TFR computed from birth rates based on MPN matching.

Proportional errors in age-specific rates based on RHH matching for American Samoa are as much as 8 percent too low at ages 15–19 and 44 percent too high at ages 44–49. Absolute errors in these rates are, of course, much smaller than the percentage errors suggest, because fertility in these extreme age groups is very low. Moreover, the errors are largely offsetting. Hence the errors in the TFR are quite small.

Illustrative analysis of the effect of mismatch on own-children fertility estimates for the United States. Mismatch also biases own-children estimates of fertility for the United States (Retherford and Cho 1978). Table 4.3 compares estimates of age-specific birth rates and TFRs derived from vital registration with parallel estimates derived by applying the own-children method to the 1970 Census. The comparison ratios in the last line of the table show a systematic age bias in the results. The own-chil-

Table 4.3. Age-specific birth rates derived alternatively from vital statistics and by applying the own-children method to the 1970 Census: United States, 1969

| | *Age group* | | | | | | | |
Derivation	*15–19*	*20–24*	*25–29*	*30–34*	*35–39*	*40–44*	*45–49*	*TFR*
Vital statistics (VS)	65.4	166.4	143.5	73.9	33.0	8.6	0.5	2,456.5
Own children (OC)	52.3	164.1	151.5	77.8	37.5	10.7	2.2	2,481.1
VS/OC	1.25	1.01	0.95	0.95	0.88	0.80	0.23	0.99

Source: Retherford and Cho (1978:573).
Note: All rates are central rates and relate to the year prior to the 1970 Census, 1 April 1969 to 1 April 1970. VS rates were obtained by weighting published rates for calendar years 1969 and 1970 by 0.75 and 0.25 respectively.

dren estimates of age-specific birth rates are too low for the 15–19 age group, about right for age groups 20–24, 25–29, and 30–34, too high beyond age 35, and increasingly so with advancing age. Overall, the bias is quite small, the comparison ratio for the total fertility rate being very close to unity.

The systematic age bias in Table 4.3 probably is due mainly to the transfer of illegitimate children of young unmarried mothers to older women with few or no children, through adoption. This is likely for two reasons. First, illegitimate births constituted nearly one-third of total births in the 15–19 age group in 1969, indicative of a high potential for adoption. Second, adopted children appear unavoidably as own children in the census, because the relationship codes do not include a separate category for adopted children.

The effect of mortality estimation errors on own-children fertility estimates

The effect of mortality estimation errors on own-children estimates of fertility has been investigated for the Republic of Korea and Thailand.

Cho (1971) employed alternative model life tables separated by five years of life expectancy to generate own-children fertility estimates for Korea, based on the 1966 Census. This work indicated that an error of five years in life expectancy introduces less than a 5 percent error in the fertility estimates, indicating a rather low level of sensitivity to mortality estimation errors.

The question of sensitivity to mortality estimation errors was subsequently investigated in more depth in an application of the own-children method to the 1970 Census of Thailand (Retherford, Chamratrithirong, and Wanglee 1980). Table 4.4 presents selected results from the analysis. Two mortality assumptions were employed: first, that mortality was the same across education categories, and second, that mortality was variable across education categories. In the first case, mortality estimates for the whole country were used. In the second case, mortality estimates by education were derived from child survivorship data (children ever born and children surviving) in the 1970 Census. The precise manner in which the mortality estimates were derived is described in the original article.

Table 4.4 shows that the maximum difference in life expectancy between education categories is about sixteen years. Life expectancy for the more educated groups is very high and may be overestimated, but such inaccuracies need not concern us here. The point to be noted is that the error in the own-children estimates of TFRs by education caused by using overall mortality in place of education-specific mortality varies between 2 percent and 8 percent, as shown in the third panel of the table. The error is smallest for those with little education, since they constitute most of the population.

Under the assumption of similar mortality across education groups, fertility differentials by education tend to be underestimated, for the following reasons: The groups with lower fertility tend also to have lower mortality. If mortality for these groups is overestimated by assuming the same mortality for all groups, then births are inflated too much by reverse survival and fertility is overestimated. Similarly, the groups with higher fertility tend also to have higher mortality. If mortality for these groups is underestimated by assuming the same mortality for all groups, then births are inflated too little by reverse survival and fertility is underestimated. The net effect is that fertility differentials by education tend to be underestimated when mortality is not specified by education. Absolute errors (the simple difference between true and estimated differential fertility) tend to be small, but relative errors (the simple difference between true and estimated differential fertility as a percentage of true) may be large.

The reason why own-children estimates of fertility tend not to be very sensitive to mortality estimation errors was alluded to in the earlier discussion of sampling variability of own-children estimates of fertility in Chapter 2. An own-children estimate of an age-specific birth rate may be viewed as the product of an age-specific child–woman ratio and a quotient of two reverse-survival ratios, one for children and the other for women. Each of these two reverse-survival ratios tends to be fairly close to one, especially when mortality is low, and the quotient of the two tends to be even closer to one. The range of variability in this quotient across different levels of mortality is rather small.

Table 4.4. Own-children fertility estimates, by women's education, based on alternative mortality assumptions: Thailand, 1965–69

Mortality assumption and ratio comparison	Education	e_0^0	TFR	Age group						
				15–19	20–24	25–29	30–34	35–39	40–44	45–49
Mortality assumption										
Same mortality across education categories	No education	66.5	6,395	143	276	293	263	195	91	18
	Some primary	66.5	6,395	90	280	305	261	213	109	21
	Some secondary	66.5	2,725	16	124	182	109	68	42	4
	Some college	66.5	1,977	1	20	130	149	59	33	5
Variable mortality across education categories	No education	63.0	6,531	146	282	300	269	199	93	18
	Some primary	66.7	6,250	88	273	298	255	208	106	20
	Some secondary	78.8	2,527	14	115	168	101	63	39	4
	Some college	78.8	1,827	1	19	120	137	54	30	4
Ratio comparison (same/variable)	No education	1.06	0.98	0.98	0.98	0.98	0.98	0.98	0.98	0.98
	Some primary	1.00	1.02	1.02	1.02	1.02	1.02	1.02	1.02	1.02
	Some secondary	0.84	1.08	1.08	1.08	1.08	1.08	1.08	1.08	1.07
	Some college	0.84	1.08	1.11	1.08	1.08	1.08	1.08	1.08	1.14

Source: Retherford, Chamratrithirong, and Wanglee (1980:8).

The effect of age misreporting on own-children fertility estimates

In most applications, age misreporting is by far the most serious source of bias in own-children estimates of fertility, particularly in less developed countries. In theory, the adjustment factors $U_{x,a}^c$ and U_a^w adjust for age misreporting as well as undercount and other kinds of misenumeration. In practice, reliable estimates of $U_{x,a}^c$ and U_a^w are rarely available. Even when they are derived from postenumeration surveys, these adjustment factors are more effective in adjusting for undercount than for age misreporting because the same kinds of age misreporting found in the original census count tend to be repeated in the postenumeration survey.

Undercount appears to be a much less serious source of error than age misreporting. A large proportion of omissions is of entire households and therefore does not necessarily have much effect on age-specific child–woman ratios, which, when adjusted for mortality, yield own-children estimates of age-specific birth rates. If the omitted households have the same composition by age and other characteristics as the included households, the omissions have no effect whatever on the own-children estimates of fertility.

Although it is probably true, as often claimed, that infants (children below one year of age) are especially prone to undercount, the frequently observed deficiency of infants in the census may stem also from age misreporting in the form of upward rounding of older infants' ages to age 1. But the apparent deficiency of children at age 0 is often less than the apparent deficiency at age 1, a pattern that could be caused by a tendency for upward rounding that is more pronounced at age 1 than at age 0. This seems a more plausible explanation than the alternative explanation that omissions are more common at age 1 than at age 0. Evidence in support of this age exaggeration hypothesis is presented later. Because of the difficulty of disentangling undercount and age misreporting, these effects are usually treated together.

Misreporting of women's ages introduces less error into the own-children estimates of fertility than misreporting of children's ages. For example, if, owing to age heaping, the census shows unusually large numbers of women aged 30, it also shows unusually large numbers of own children of mothers aged 30. Because children are matched to mothers, heaping of mothers' ages on 30, even when severe, does not radically distort corresponding age-specific child–woman ratios, so that women of reported ages 29, 30, and 31 have about the same child–woman ratios as would have been observed had there been no age misreporting at all. As discussed in the next chapter, misreporting of women's ages can still

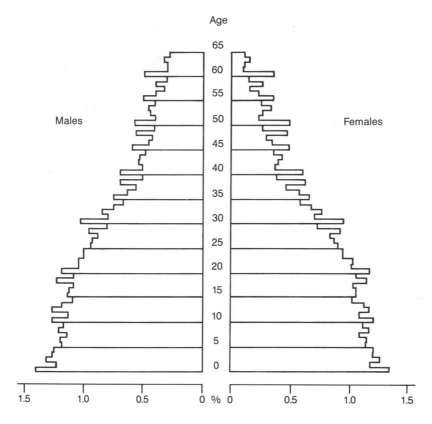

Figure 4.3. Age pyramid derived from the 1981 Census: Sri Lanka

Source: Ratnayake, Retherford, and Sivasubramaniam (1984:4).

produce systematic distortions in the overall age pattern of fertility, but the effect on the total fertility rate tends to be small.

Misreporting of children's ages is another matter. It has more serious consequences because it can produce large overestimates of fertility in some calendar years and large underestimates in others. Heaping on age 5, for example, inflates fertility estimates for the sixth year previous to the census, which is the birth year of children aged 5 at the time of the census.

To check for the presence of age misreporting, one should always begin by plotting an age pyramid by single years of age. An illustrative example for Sri Lanka in 1981 is shown in Figure 4.3. The figure shows some evidence of heaping on ages ending in 0 and 5, which helps explain some of the year-to-year fluctuations observed in the derived TFR trend, shown before in Figure 2.2. Myers's index of digit preference (Shryock and Siegel 1973:206ff.) provides a numerical measure of age heaping that is also useful.

Another check involves comparison of fertility estimates derived from own children with fertility estimates derived from vital registration. Fertility estimates derived from vital registration are not affected at all by heaping of children's ages, since births are registered directly, whereas own-children estimates of fertility show peaks and troughs in certain calendar years according to the pattern of heaping of children's ages in the census. Such comparisons therefore tend to reveal the effects of misreporting of children's ages in the census. Figure 4.4 shows such a comparison for Japan, where the agreement between the two sets of estimates is excellent. The agreement would be even better if calendar years lined up more precisely. The midpoint of calendar years is July for the vital statistics estimates and April for the own-children estimates. The discrepancy of three months affects the magnitude of the fertility dip in 1966. This fertility dip stems from the widespread belief that the Chinese Zodiacal Year of the Fire Horse (in this case, 1966) is not propitious for childbearing. The year 1966 from vital statistics coincides precisely with the Year of the Fire Horse, whereas the year 1966 from the own-children analysis includes only nine months of the Year of the Fire Horse, and that is why the fertility dip derived from vital statistics is more pronounced than the dip derived by the own-children method.

Of course, as the above example illustrates, the discrepancies revealed by such comparisons may indicate errors other than age misreporting. Another example is the previous comparison in Table 4.3, which revealed mismatch of adopted children. Another difficulty is that populations with severe age misreporting in censuses tend also to have deficient vital registration. In such cases comparisons of fertility estimates derived from own-children data with fertility estimates derived from vital registration may test the completeness of vital registration more than they test the accuracy of the own-children estimates of fertility. In applications of the own-children method in island populations in the South Pacific, for example, it has been found that fertility estimates derived from own-children data almost invariably exceed fertility estimates derived from vital registration. The discrepancies suggest underregistration of births (Levin and Retherford 1986).

In other types of demographic analysis, smoothing techniques are often used to eliminate or reduce the effects of age misreporting. These must be used cautiously in own-children analysis because age misreporting causes not only annual fluctuations in the own-children estimates of

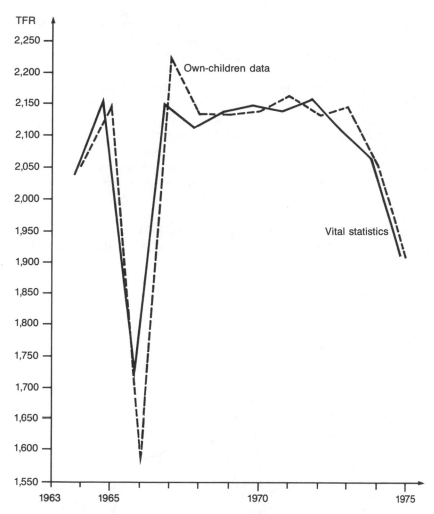

Figure 4.4. Estimated total fertility rates derived alternatively from census data on own children and vital registration data: Japan, 1964–75

Source: Itoh (1981).

fertility but also systematic distortions in the long-term trend and overall age pattern of fertility. Smoothing techniques tend to eliminate year-to-year fluctuations, but they are usually ineffective in eliminating bias in long-term trends and overall age patterns. In practice, the detailed, unsmoothed estimates may provide useful clues about how age misreporting biases the long-term trends and overall age patterns of estimated fertility. Premature smoothing of the data eliminates these clues and restricts possibilities of analysis of errors. To the extent that smoothing is attempted, it should be done only after an initial examination of the detailed unsmoothed estimates. The preferred method of smoothing is simple aggregation for groups of ages (typically five-year age groups) and groups of calendar years, as described in previous chapters.

Experience in applying the own-children method in many populations suggests that a sufficient level of initial detail in the tabulations of own-children estimates of fertility is five-year age groups and one-year time periods. The age-specific birth rates in five-year age groups and the TFR should each be graphed against time in single calendar years, as in Figure 4.5, which is an illustrative graph of the TFR trend in Pakistan, based on the 1973 Housing, Economic, and Demographic Survey (HED). In this case, the plot by single calendar years shows clear evidence of age misreporting. Figure 4.5 shows major fertility peaks in the ninth, eleventh, and thirteenth years before the survey, corresponding to children of ages

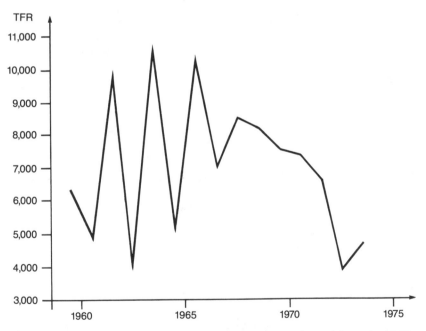

Figure 4.5. Own-children estimates of total fertility rates derived from the 1973 Housing, Economic, and Demographic Survey: Pakistan, 1959–73

Source: Retherford et al. (1985:19).

8, 10, and 12 at the time of the survey. Since Pakistan censuses and surveys are noted for major heaping on ages 8, 10, and 12, one suspects that the trend in the TFR is severely biased by age misreporting.

When results from just one census or survey are available, it is very difficult to distinguish spurious trends and age patterns of fertility from real trends and age patterns. Results from two or more censuses enable a more definitive analysis. For example, if own-children estimates of fertility are available from two censuses taken ten years apart, each census yields a fifteen-year fertility trend, and the two trends overlap during the five years immediately preceding the first of the two censuses. If each trend is spuriously distorted in the same way by age misreporting (and perhaps other sources of systematic bias as well), the two trends will overlap poorly, and each will show the same pattern of distortion. The spurious aspects of the trend will be apparent, and it may be possible to discern approximately the true trend from the comparison. An extended example of this kind of analysis, focusing on Pakistan, is presented in Chapter 5.

If own-children estimates of fertility are available from several successive censuses, own-children estimates of cohort fertility can be checked against reported numbers of children ever born. Suppose, for example, that the own-children method has been applied to censuses taken in 1960, 1970, and 1980, yielding a set of age-specific birth rates for every year between 1945 and 1979. Recall from Chapter 2 that the own-children method yields period–cohort age-specific birth rates as well as central (age–period) age-specific birth rates, and that the period–cohort age-specific birth rates can be chained together along cohort corridors in the Lexis diagram to estimate age-specific fertility for real cohorts. For a given cohort, these period–cohort age-specific birth rates can be cumulated to estimate mean numbers of children ever born at specified ages of women, and these own-children estimates of children ever born at a specified age can be compared with children ever born for the same cohort of women at the same age as reported directly in a particular census. Such comparisons can be distorted by in- and out-migration, so that this test is a global test for many kinds of errors, not just age misreporting.

Figure 4.6 shows an example for the state of Wisconsin in the United States (Retherford and Sewell 1986). Period–cohort rates for the real cohort of ages 28–31 in 1970 and ages 38–41 in 1980 were reconstructed by applying the own-children method to the 1970 and 1980 censuses. The cohort's average age was, to a close approximation, exactly 30 in 1970 and exactly 40 in 1980, and we view the cohort as concentrated at these two ages at these two dates. Three age-specific birth rates (ASBRs) for this cohort can be derived from the 1970 Census: an ASBR at 15–19 for 1955–59, an ASBR at 20–24 for 1960–64, and an ASBR at 25–29 for 1965–69. Likewise, three age-specific birth rates can be derived from the 1980 Census: an ASBR at 25–29 for 1965–69, an ASBR at 30–34 for 1970–74,and as ASBR at 35–39 for 1975–79. The calculations are all done initially by single years of age, with numerators and denominators aggregated separately over age and time before they are divided to get period–cohort age-specific rates in five-year age groups over five-year time periods. The ASBRs at 25–29 for 1965–69 overlap, and in general they will not agree. (Note the discontinuity at 25–29 in Figure 4.6; the discontinuity is large in Panel A and negligible in Panel B.) The final estimate of the ASBR at 25–29 for 1965–69 may be taken as the average of the two.

If the final set of ASBRs for 15–19, 20–24, . . ., 35–39 is totaled and the sum multiplied by five, the result is an estimate of cumulative fertility per woman at exact age 40 in 1980. This estimate can be compared with the mean number of reported children even born at exact age 40 in 1980. An estimate of the mean number of children ever born at exact age 40 is obtained by averaging the reported number of children ever born at ages 38, 39, 40, and 41. The own-children estimate of cumulative fertility and the estimated mean number of children ever born should agree. In the case of high school dropouts in Figure 4.6, the respective values of cumulative fertility and children ever born at exact age 40 are 3.39 and 3.46, which agree to within 2.0 percent (with children ever born taken as the base). In the case of high school graduates (those with twelve completed years of education), the respective values of cumulative fertility and children ever born at exact age 40 are 3.15 and 2.99, which agree to within 5.3 percent.

Errors in fertility estimates by characteristics that change over the adult life cycle

As mentioned earlier, one strength of the own-children method that enhances its usefulness in more developed as well as less developed countries is that it allows tabulation of fertility estimates by socioeconomic characteristics such as education. It is important to note, however, that the method treats demographic characteristics such as age, parity, and duration since first marriage differently than it treats socioeconomic characteristics such as income or labor force activity status. When own-children estimates of fertility are tabulated by age, parity, or duration since first marriage, these characteristics describe women during the year for which fertility is being estimated, some years before the census. But

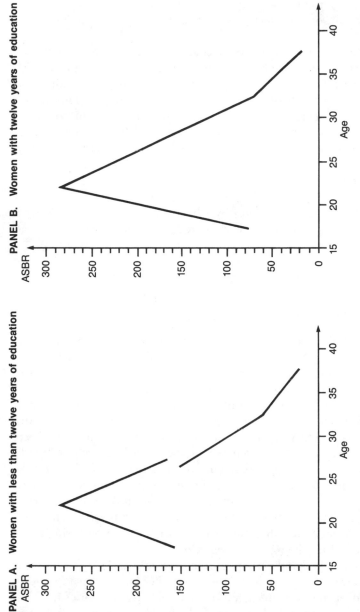

Figure 4.6. Period–cohort age-specific birth rates, by education, for the cohort of women aged 28–31 in the 1970 U.S. Census and 38–41 in the 1980 U.S. Census: Wisconsin

Source: Based on unpublished tabulations from Public Use Sample tapes from the 1970 and 1980 censuses.

Note: Women with more than twelve years of education are not shown.

when the estimates are tabulated by socioeconomic characteristics such as income or labor force activity status, these characteristics describe women at the time of the census, not during the year for which fertility is being estimated.

Problems arise with socioeconomic characteristics such as income and labor force activity status, which tend to change over the adult life cycle. The difficulty is that, say, income may be quite different for an individual at the time of the census from what it was a few years earlier. This means that, for a period several years before a census, the own-children estimates of fertility by income may differ substantially from independently derived estimates of fertility by income where in the latter instance income pertains to the year in question rather than the time of the census. In this situation, the own-children estimates of fertility by income can be misleading.

Own-children fertility estimates by labor force activity status derived from the 1980 Census of Japan (Kawasaki 1985: table 3) provide a dramatic illustration:

Status	*1970*	*1975*	*1980*
Employed	2.115	1.671	0.896
Not employed	2.187	2.237	2.831

They indicate a sharp decline in the fertility of employed women and a sharp increase in the fertility of women who were not employed. These results are highly misleading. Were it possible to tabulate the fertility estimates in this table by activity status at the time the births actually occurred rather than at the time of the census, the results would have been quite different. Only slight changes in fertility by activity status would have been indicated, and they would not necessarily have been even in the same direction, much less at the same level, as the trends shown in the table. The apparent but spurious decline in the TFR of employed women in the table occurs because some women who were employed at the time of the census in 1980, and thus unlikely to be caring for an infant at that time, were not employed five or ten years before the census in 1975 or 1970, when they were more likely to be caring for a baby by virtue of not being employed. Conversely, some of the women who were unemployed and perhaps caring for a baby in 1980, at the time of the census, were employed in 1975 or 1970. Because of these compositional shifts over time within each of the two activity categories in Table 4.5, the TFR falls sharply but spuriously for the employed and rises sharply but spuriously for the unemployed. For further illustration and discussion of effects of this kind, see Rindfuss (1977).

If the own-children method is used to tabulate fertility trends by characteristics that change significantly over the adult life cycle, it is clear that the results must be interpreted cautiously. The estimated trends are of more methodological than substantive interest. Of course, the distinction between characteristics that change and those that do not is not always clear-cut. In the case of education, for example, those who go on for higher education experience changes in educational status for a few years after the beginning of the reproductive period, thereby muddying somewhat the interpretation of fertility trends by education. On the whole, however, educational attainment changes little over the adult life cycle.

Although the estimates of fertility trends by characteristics that change over the adult life cycle may be severely biased, it is still reasonably valid to make fertility comparisons across the categories of such a variable if attention is confined to the first year before the census. If such tabulations are made from more than one census, the results usually yield reliable estimates of trends.

CHAPTER 5

Illustrative Evaluations of Own-Children Fertility Estimates for Korea and Pakistan

This chapter elaborates a number of points made in earlier chapters. Two illustrative analyses are presented, one for the Republic of Korea and the other for Pakistan.

Korea

The own-children method has been applied extensively in Korea, with good results. Age is reckoned according to the zodiacal animal year of birth in Korea, and, because people know the animal associated with their year of birth, ages are reported very accurately. Therefore, bias due to age misreporting in the own-children estimates of fertility is usually minimal. Sometimes, however, there have been problems in accurately converting age as reckoned in the traditional lunar calendar system to age as reckoned in the Western system (Coale, Cho, and Goldman 1980). Two extended examples are considered, the first involving own-children estimates of fertility by age only, and the second involving own-children estimates of fertility by duration since first marriage.

Own-children fertility estimates by age. The accuracy of own-children estimates of fertility by age has been evaluated by comparing overlapping estimates fertility trends, derived alternatively from the 1975 and 1980 censuses and the 1974 Korean National Fertility Survey (KNFS), which was part of the World Fertility Survey (Retherford, Cho, and Kim 1983). Figures 5.1 and 5.2 summarize the results of this analysis.

Figure 5.1 compares annual estimates of total fertility rates for 1966–80 derived from the 1980 Census with overlapping estimates for 1966–75 derived from the 1975 Census and with estimates for 1966–74 derived from the 1974 KNFS. The three sets of estimates are in very close agreement, especially from 1972 onward. All three sources indicate that the decline of fertility was interrupted by a temporary rise during the late 1960s. The 1980 Census and the KNFS indicate a larger rise than does the 1975 Census, and the 1980 Census indicates a peak in 1969, whereas the 1975 Census and the KNFS indicate a peak in 1971. But these discrepancies are minor, as is visually apparent from the figure.

Figure 5.2 compares annual estimates of age-specific birth rates derived from the same three data sources. Again the agreement is very good. The KNFS estimates show a somewhat more jagged pattern than the census estimates (true of the overall TFR estimates in Figure 5.1 as well), and this probably stems from greater sampling variability due to a much smaller sample size. The KNFS estimates tend to be somewhat higher than the census estimates at ages 25–29, 35–39, and 40–44 and somewhat lower at ages 15–19, but these differences are slight.

Figure 5.2 also shows that the increase in total fertility during the late 1960s, shown in Figure 5.1, stemmed from increases in age-specific birth rates at ages 20–34 and especially at ages 25–29. At ages below 20 and over 35 fertility rates declined over the entire period, except for a hint of an increase during the late 1960s at ages 35–39.

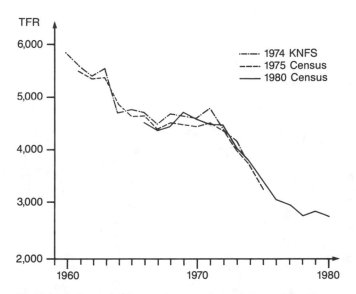

Figure 5.1. Own-children estimates of trends in total fertility rates derived from the 1974 Korean National Fertility Survey and the 1975 and 1980 censuses: Republic of Korea, 1960–80

Source: Retherford, Cho, and Kim (1983:13).

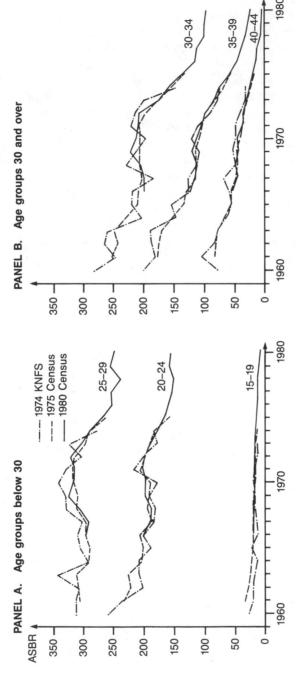

Figure 5.2. Own-children estimates of trends in age-specific birth rates derived from the 1974 Korean National Fertility Survey and the 1975 and 1980 censuses: Republic of Korea, 1960–80

Source: Retherford, Cho, and Kim (1983:13).

Own-children fertility estimates by duration since first marriage. The methodology for extending the own-children method by using data on duration since first marriage was originally tested for Cheju Province, based on data from the 1975 Census (Cho and Retherford 1978). A more extensive test, comparing overlapping estimates derived alternatively from the 1975 and 1980 censuses, employed data for the entire country (Retherford, Cho, and Kim 1984).

The analysis began with a comparison of fertility estimates derived from pregnancy histories with fertility estimates derived from own children, based on data from the 1974 KNFS. The KNFS was used because it is widely regarded as a survey of good quality and because it contains an individual sample with maternity histories embedded in a large household sample, allowing application of both methods to essentially the same data set. Table 5.1 shows estimates of age-specific and duration-specific ever-marital birth rates computed for 1963–67 and 1968–72 using each method, with comparison ratios in the fourth and seventh columns. The comparison ratios are generally close to one, except at ages 15–19 and durations 0 and 1, where discrepancies are mostly in the 10 to 20 percent range. These latter discrepancies are probably due to data errors, apparently introduced in the editing process and currently being investigated, that affect proportions married computed from the KNFS household tape (Retherford and Alam 1985).

The rates derived from the KNFS for 1968–1972 are graphed in Figures 5.3 and 5.4 along with comparable own-children estimates derived from the 1975 and 1980 censuses. The four sets of estimates of age-specific ever-marital birth rates in Figure 5.3 agree closely at ages above 25. The agreement at ages 20–24 is also rather good, but at ages 15–19 there is considerable disagreement. Own-children estimates based on the KNFS give the highest estimate at ages 15–19, and own-children estimates based on the 1975 Census give the lowest estimate.

The discrepancies are rather surprising, because age-specific birth rates for all women estimated from the KNFS and the 1975 and 1980 censuses show good agreement at all ages, as seen in the previous section. It is also surprising that ever-marital fertility is consistently lower at ages 15–19 than at ages 20–24. The downturn at ages 15–19 is inconsistent with estimates of fertility for currently married women (obtained by dividing own-children estimates of age-specific fertility for all women by proportions currently married at the same age), which show considerably higher fertility for currently married women at 15–19 than at 20–24. The estimates of fertility for currently married women (marital fertility) at 15–19 are on the order of 450–500 per thousand, compared with 300–400 in Figure 5.3 (Cho and Retherford 1986). On the assumption of no illegiti-

Table 5.1. Age-specific and duration-specific ever-marital birth rates derived from the 1974 Korean National Fertility Survey: Republic of Korea, 1963–67 and 1968–72

Age group or duration	1963–67			1968–72		
	Pregnancy history (PH)	Own-children (OC)	PH/OC	Pregnancy history (PH)	Own-children (OC)	PH/OC
Age						
15–19	291	333	0.87	328	410	0.80
20–24	363	370	0.98	402	423	0.95
25–29	327	326	1.00	357	358	1.00
30–34	231	222	1.04	213	219	0.97
35–39	—	—	—	111	110	1.01
Duration						
0	310	403	0.77	415	489	0.85
1	486	417	1.17	448	458	0.98
2	311	339	0.92	400	395	1.01
3	371	351	1.06	416	395	1.05
4	338	343	0.99	344	355	0.97
5	337	340	0.99	340	336	1.01
6	316	314	1.01	329	327	1.01
7	316	304	1.04	313	313	1.00
8	303	286	1.06	276	281	0.98
9	253	266	0.95	229	259	0.88
10	—	—	—	258	238	1.08
11	—	—	—	219	220	1.00
12	—	—	—	179	193	0.93
13	—	—	—	170	169	1.01
14	—	—	—	148	161	0.92

Source: Retherford, Cho, and Kim (1984:541).
Notes: The KNFS household schedule collected information on age at first marriage only for ever-married women below age 50. Because women aged 50 at the time of the survey were 44 in 1968 and 39 in 1963, OC estimates for five-year age groups must be truncated at age 40 for the period of 1968–72 and at age 35 for the period 1963–67 to avoid bias and achieve comparability with census-based estimates. Since virtually all women in Korea who ever marry do so by age 30, OC duration-specific birth rates for 1968–72 are biased for durations above 9, and rates for 1963–67 are biased for durations above 14. Rates for those durations are not shown in this table. Pregnancy history estimates are compared with own-children estimates. Both sets of estimates are based on the 1974 KNFS.

mate fertility, ever-marital fertility and marital fertility should agree closely because at ages 15–19 the number of ever married women is virtually identical to the number of currently married women. The divergence between ever-marital fertility and marital fertility suggests either an implausibly high level of illegitimate fertility or some kind of systematic

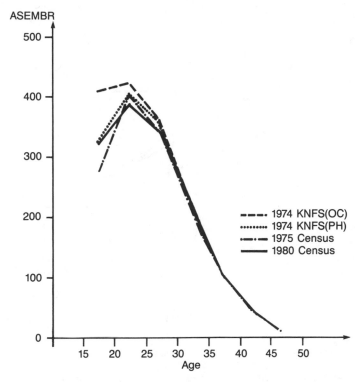

Figure 5.3. Age-specific ever-marital birth rates for the period 1968–72, estimated alternatively by applying the own-children method to the 1974 Korea National Fertility Survey and the 1975 and 1980 censuses, and by applying the pregnancy history method to the 1974 Korean National Fertility Survey: Republic of Korea

Source: Retherford, Cho, and Kim (1984:542).

Note: PH denotes the pregnancy history method and OC denotes the own-children method. Because of truncation problems (see text), KNFS values for ages 40 and over are omitted.

error in the data. The discrepancies in Figure 5.3 and further evidence presented below suggest that the latter possibility is more plausible than the former.

In Figure 5.4 three of the four sets of estimates of duration-specific ever-marital birth rates agree rather well, except at durations 0 and 1. Estimates based on the 1975 Census, however, differ strikingly from the other three sets and appear consistently to underestimate fertility at every

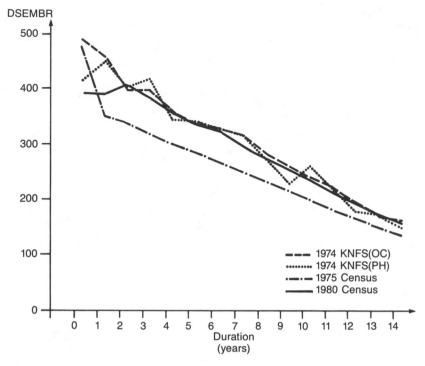

Figure 5.4. Duration-specific ever-marital birth rates for the period 1968–72, estimated alternatively by applying the own-children method to the 1974 Korean National Fertility Survey and the 1975 and 1980 censuses, and by applying the pregnancy history method to the 1974 Korean National Fertility Survey: Republic of Korea

Source: Retherford, Cho, and Kim (1984:543).

duration except 0. Note that the curves are smoother for the census-based estimates than for the KNFS-based estimates, which are based on a much smaller sample.

Figures 5.5 and 5.6 shed additional light on the discrepancies revealed in Figures 5.3 and 5.4 by showing how well trends in ever-marital total fertility rates $EMTFR_a$ and $EMTFR_d$, estimated alternatively from the 1975 and 1980 censuses, agree during the 1966–75 period of overlapping trends. The overlap for $EMTFR_a$ is rather good, but that for $EMTFR_d$ is poor, with estimates derived from the 1975 Census again consistently lower than those derived from the 1980 Census, except during the first three years of the overlap period.

Figures 5.7 and 5.8, which examine overlap in age-specific and dura-

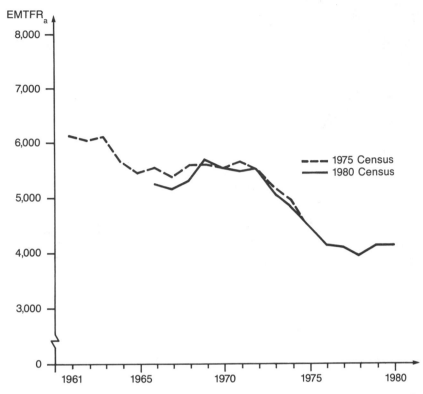

Figure 5.5. Trends in EMTFR$_a$ derived from the 1975 and 1980 censuses: Republic Korea, 1961–80

Source: Retherford, Cho, and Kim (1984:544).

tion-specific ever-marital birth rates, provide further detail. Figure 5.7 shows that trends in age-specific rates overlap closely for ages over 25 and fairly closely for rates at ages 20–24, but quite poorly for rates at ages 15–19. The divergence at 15–19 is systematic but difficult to interpret, especially since it involves a crossover. (Recall that the discrepancies at ages 15–19 do not affect EMTFR$_a$, which excludes fertility in this age group.) Figure 5.8 shows a much more striking lack of good overlap of trends in duration-specific birth rates. Estimates derived from the 1975 Census are consistently lower than estimates derived from the 1980 Census at all durations except 0, where the discrepancy is reversed.

The rather good agreement between estimates derived from the 1980 Census and those derived from the 1974 KNFS suggests that the principal source of divergence between estimates derived alternatively from the

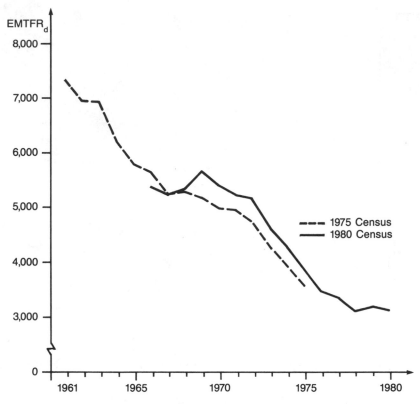

Figure 5.6. Trends in EMTFR$_d$ derived from the 1975 and 1980 censuses: Republic of Korea, 1961–80

Source: Retherford, Cho, and Kim (1984:545).

1975 and 1980 censuses is data errors in the 1975 Census. In addition, the fact that ever-marital fertility estimates derived from the 1975 and 1980 censuses agree better when specified by age only than when specified by duration only suggests that the root of the problem may lie in the quality of the 1975 data on age at first marriage from which duration was calculated.

Indeed, the observed discrepancies in ever-marital fertility estimates are consistent with the hypothesis that in the 1975 Census age was recorded correctly but that age at first marriage was not converted accurately from the traditional Korean system of age reckoning into the Western system, which is used in census tabulation. On one hand, it is likely that current age was converted fairly accurately into the Western system,

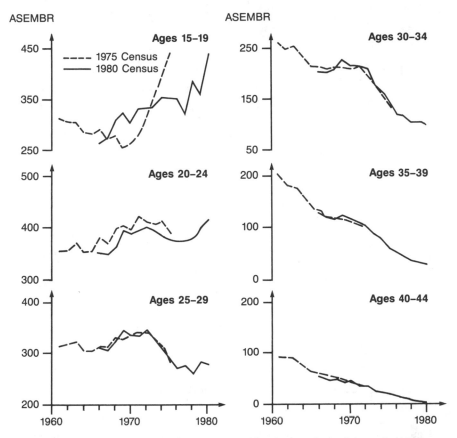

Figure 5.7. Trends in age-specific ever-marital birth rates derived from the 1975 and 1980 censuses: Republic of Korea, 1961–80

Source: Retherford, Cho, and Kim (1984:547).

for two reasons: first, because fifteen years earlier improper conversion of current age had posed difficult problems for those analyzing the 1960 Census and those problems had been satisfactorily resolved in the 1966 Census; and second, because patterns of age-specific birth rates and age-specific ever-marital birth rates, estimated alternatively from different data sources, are reasonably consistent (Retherford, Cho, and Kim 1983; also Figures 5.5 and 5.6 in this chapter). On the other hand, mistakes may have been made in converting age at first marriage into the Western system in 1975, since the 1975 Census was the first Korean census to ask age at first marriage.

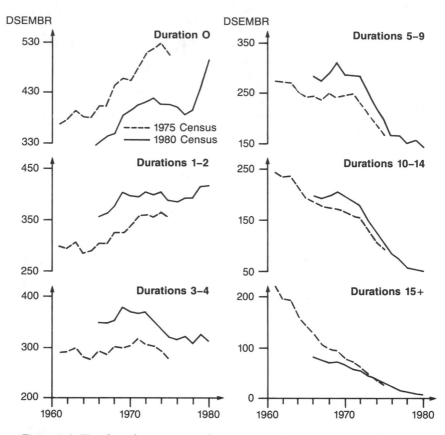

Figure 5.8. Trends in duration-specific ever-marital birth rates derived from the 1975 and 1980 censuses: Republic of Korea, 1961–80

Source: Retherford, Cho, and Kim (1984:548).

Suppose that age at first marriage was recorded in the traditional Korean system instead of the Western system of age reckoning in a high proportion of cases in the 1975 Census but not in the 1980 Census. In the traditional system, a child is counted as one year of age when he or she is born and advances one year of age every subsequent January 1. If age is given in the Western system and age at first marriage in the traditional system, then marriage duration, which is computed as the difference between current age and age at marriage, will be too short. That is, someone who is assigned to, say, duration 3, may be actually duration 4 or even duration 5. Since fertility declines by duration, this means that the estimated birth rate for duration 3 will be lower than it should be.

This is indeed the pattern we observe for the 1975 census-derived estimates at durations above 0 in Figure 5.8.

But what about the reversal at duration 0? If the above reasoning is correct, it is plausible that a bunching of births occurs at duration 0. If reported duration 3 is really duration 4, then reported duration 0 is really duration 1, and reported duration −1 is really duration 0. But duration −1 means an illegitimate birth, which in many cases the interviewer probably noticed and surmised was not correct. In such instances the interviewer may have probed and ended by revising the recorded age at marriage so that births that might otherwise have been reported as duration −1 were reported as duration 0 instead. The consequent bunching of births at duration 0 could then produce an overestimate rather than underestimate of fertility at duration 0.

Of course, in many instances interviewers undoubtedly did not perceive the implication of illegitimacy. Hence one expects spuriously high numbers of illegitimate births at the younger reproductive ages. The data in Table 5.2 confirm this expectation. The table compares 1975 and 1980 Census estimates of births to never-married women as a percentage of total births in each age group. (Total births in each age group were computed by means of the original version of the own-children method, which estimates fertility by age only.) The percentages derived from the 1975 Census are much higher than those derived from the 1980 Census. At the younger reproductive ages these apparently illegitimate births are concentrated at 15–19 and to a lesser extent at 20–24, the two age groups in which most marriages occur. Percentages at these ages show a slight tendency to decrease down columns as the census enumeration date is approached, which is plausible, because an enumerator is more likely to perceive the implication of illegitimacy for younger women and younger children than for older women and older children. (The mental subtraction of age at marriage from current age is easier in the case of younger women because the difference between these two ages is smaller for younger women than for older women; likewise, subtractions involving children's ages are easier if the children are infants or very young.) Of course, with increased availability of contraception and abortion, it is possible that illegitimacy actually did decrease over the period.

Table 5.2 also shows a second concentration of illegitimate births at the older reproductive ages in the case of the 1975 Census estimates but not at all in the 1980 Census. This finding suggests that in the 1975 Census many older remarried women erroneously reported a second marriage as a first marriage. Children by the first marriage then appear to be illegitimate. Perhaps other errors are also implicated, since the percentages in the upper right of this table are surprisingly high. The likely rea-

Table 5.2. Own-children estimates of births to never-married women as a percentage of total births in each specified age group, derived from the 1975 and 1980 censuses: Republic of Korea, 1961–80

Census and year	Age group						
	15–19	20–24	25–29	30–34	35–39	40–44	45–49
1975 Census							
1961	37	11	2	15	62	75	74
1962	36	11	2	8	55	72	73
1963	39	13	2	4	43	69	78
1964	43	12	2	2	30	65	68
1965	39	13	2	1	22	59	64
1966	37	13	3	0	13	53	62
1967	35	14	3	0	7	40	54
1968	39	17	4	0	3	31	54
1969	41	17	4	0	2	23	48
1970	36	18	4	0	0	16	47
1971	37	18	4	0	0	10	44
1972	36	17	4	0	0	4	29
1973	32	16	4	0	0	1	20
1974	28	14	4	0	0	1	27
1975	33	17	5	0	0	0	17
1980 Census							
1966	22	4	1	0	0	0	0
1967	23	5	1	0	0	0	0
1968	23	6	1	0	0	0	0
1969	24	5	1	0	0	0	0
1970	25	5	1	0	0	0	0
1971	18	5	1	0	0	0	0
1972	21	5	1	0	0	0	0
1973	21	6	1	0	0	0	0
1974	18	5	1	0	0	0	0
1975	15	5	1	0	0	0	0
1976	13	4	1	0	0	0	0
1977	15	4	1	0	0	0	0
1978	11	5	1	0	0	0	0
1979	15	5	1	0	0	0	0
1980	0	0	0	0	0	0	0

Source: Retherford, Cho, and Kim (1984:550).
Note: Births to never-married women in each age group were obtained as the difference between births to all women, derived by the original own-children method, and births to ever-married women, derived by the extended own-children method.

son why percentages decline sharply as one reads down the last three columns of the upper panel of the table is that the probability that a child is from a previous marriage increases with age of child. (Recall that birth rates for years near the census data are based on young children and that rates for years further back in time are based on older children.)

Details about how the question on age at first marriage was asked in 1975 and 1980 support the above reasoning. In 1975 no clear distinction was made between first marriages and second marriages in the question on age at marriage. Moreover, the question did not make clear whether age was being asked in the traditional lunar calendar system or the Western system. Year and month of marriage were also asked, distinguishing traditional and Western reporting, but apparently this information was not used effectively to refine the estimate of marriage age.

These problems were corrected in the 1980 Census. Age at marriage was asked in the Korean system and converted to Western age by established procedures, and care was taken to specify that the marriage in question was the first marriage. Table 5.2 suggests, however, that reporting was still not perfect in 1980. Statistics on illegitimacy are not available to provide an independent check, but the illegitimacy ratios derived from the 1980 Census still seem implausibly high. Illegitimacy meets with considerable social disapproval in Korea, and illegitimacy ratios are believed to be low. Moreover, the illegitimacy ratio's sudden drop to 0 in 1980 in the bottom row of the table is suspect. It almost certainly stems from data problems, not to a sudden decline in illegitimate fertility.

Table 5.3 provides additional evidence that age at marriage was misreported in the 1975 Census. The table compares 1975 and 1980 census estimates of mean age at marriage for five-year age cohorts of women who were at least 30 years old in 1975. In the first row of the table, for example, the mean age at marriage for those 30–34 in 1975 is compared with the mean age at marriage for those 35–39 in 1980. This comparison is legitimate as long as there were no further marriages in the cohort between 1975 and 1980, and as long as cohort attrition from mortality and migration was not selective by age at first marriage. The first condition is approximately met, since about 98 percent of Korean women marry by age 30 (Cho and Retherford 1986). We have no evidence regarding attrition selectivity by age at marriage, but it is probably negligible. The comparisons show that estimates of mean age at first marriage derived from the 1975 Census are 0.4–0.7 year higher than corresponding estimates derived from the 1980 Census. The discrepancy is in the expected direction. Note that without the few additional marriages that occurred in each cohort between 1975 and 1980, the differences in Table

Table 5.3. Mean age at marriage for four
cohorts of women, derived from the 1975 and
1980 censuses: Republic of Korea

Cohort age in 1975	Census on which estimate is based		Difference
	1975	1980	
30–34	22.1	21.7	0.4
35–39	21.5	20.9	0.6
40–44	20.8	20.2	0.6
45–49	19.8	19.1	0.7

Source: Retherford, Cho, and Kim (1984:551).

5.3 would have been even larger. The additional marriages work to
increase the mean age at marriage, but Table 5.3 shows decreases.

The slope of the curve in Figure 5.4 (birth rates by duration) implies
that an average error of 0.4–0.7 year in estimated duration causes an
error in the estimated birth rate at a given duration of only about 10 per
thousand at most durations. But the discrepancies between the estimates
derived alternatively from the two censuses are usually considerably
greater than this. The explanation of this inconsistency is unclear, and it
suggests that the explanation of the discrepancies is incomplete.

Misreporting of age at marriage in the 1975 Census helps also to
explain why discrepancies in age-specific ever-marital birth rates derived
alternatively from the 1975 and 1980 censuses are substantial only at
15–19 and, to a much lesser extent, at 20–24. These are the ages at
which most women marry and therefore the ages at which births erroneously classified as illegitimate are concentrated. The exclusion of these
births from ever-marital birth rates helps to explain why the estimates of
ever-marital fertility at ages 15–19, relative to estimates at 20–24, are
lower than expected in Figure 5.3.

A puzzling feature of Figure 5.8 is that birth rates for durations 15+
are not much lower than those for durations 10–14 for the early 1960s,
when estimated from the 1975 Census. One expects the rate for durations 15+ to be considerably lower than that for durations 10–14, as is
true of the estimates derived from the 1980 Census.

On the whole, the own-children method appears to give quite accurate
estimates of fertility for Korea. In the case of own-children estimates of
fertility by duration, however, results are sensitive to systematic error in
converting age from the traditional lunar system to the Western system.

The analysis demonstrates that application of the own-children method to two or more censuses or surveys provides overlapping estimates of fertility trends that can be used to track down the errors.

Pakistan

The initial application of the own-children method in Pakistan was to the 1973 Housing, Economic, and Demographic (HED) Survey (Retherford and Mirza 1982). The sampling frame for this survey consisted of enumeration blocks from the 100 percent census enumeration of 1972. Approximately 2 percent of rural households and 5 percent of urban households were selected from the full 1972 count for reinterview with a longer questionnaire. The Pakistan data are characterized by severe age misreporting and pose estimation problems quite different from those encountered in the Korean application.

The complete single-year age pyramid from the HED Survey (not shown) indicates extensive heaping of women's ages on years ending in 0 and 5. Children's ages show extensive heaping on 8, 10, and 12, as shown in Figure 5.9. The figure includes children's age distributions not only from the HED Survey, but also from the 1968 and 1972 Population Growth Surveys and the 1972 Census, which show a similar pattern. Note that these age distributions of children are, approximately, a mirror image of the TFR trend derived from the HED Survey, shown in Figure 4.5. Together, Figures 4.5 and 5.9 suggest that the TFR trend in Figure 4.5 may be completely spurious and that in fact the TFR may have been approximately constant over the estimation period.

Not only the trend but also the age pattern of fertility derived by applying the own-children method to the HED Survey is biased. It appears that age heaping of women is systematically biased upward, in the form of age exaggeration that increases with age. In early research on the HED Survey, it was thought that this patten of age exaggeration could explain the implausible age pattern of fertility change, shown in Table 5.4, whereby estimated marital fertility undergoes substantial percentage increases at the younger reproductive ages and substantial percentage declines at the older reproductive ages, with monotonically declining percentage changes at intermediate ages.

On one hand, the apparent fall in marital fertility at the older reproductive ages could be real if the practice of family limitation were rapidly taking hold in the population. But comparison of rates of contraceptive use from the National Impact Survey of 1968–69 and the Pakistan Fertility Survey of 1975 offers no evidence that family limitation has taken

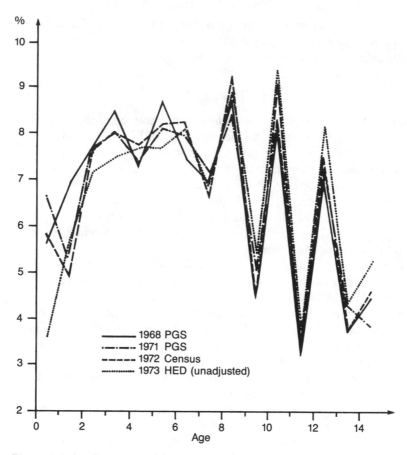

Figure 5.9. Single-year age distribution of the population aged 0–14: Pakistan, various dates and sources

Source: Retherford and Mirza (1982:259).

Note: PGS denotes Population Growth Survey; HED, Housing, Economic, and Demographic Survey.

hold in any significant portion of the population. On the other hand, older women's ages might be increasingly exaggerated as age increases. The potential for such exaggeration is great. Judged from the amount of age heaping in the 1972 Census and the 1973 HED Survey, few women in Pakistan know their birth date accurately. In the Pakistan Fertility Survey of 1975, only 6 percent of women knew their birth date; either the respondent or the interviewer had to make an educated guess for the remaining 94 percent.

Table 5.4. Own-children estimates of total fertility rates, age-specific birth rates, standardized marital general fertility rates, and age-specific marital birth rates, derived from the 1973 Housing, Economic, and Demographic Survey: Pakistan, 1962–66 and 1967–71

Rate and age group	1962–66	1967–71	% change
Fertility			
15–19	142	149	4.9
20–24	290	324	11.6
25–29	305	328	7.5
30–34	276	280	1.4
35–39	217	209	–4.0
40–44	153	143	–6.7
45–49	101	86	–14.3
TFR	7,423	7,592	2.3
Marital fertility			
15–19	295	366	23.9
20–24	345	401	16.3
25–29	332	358	8.0
30–34	296	299	1.2
35–39	237	225	–5.1
40–44	178	162	–8.9
45–49	122	101	–16.9
SMGFR	253	262	3.6

Source: Retherford and Mirza (1982:260).
Note: SMGFR denotes the standardized marital general fertility rate, calculated as $\Sigma_a P_{sa} F_a$, where the summation ranges over ages 15–49 in five-year age groups, F_a denotes the age-specific marital birth rates at ages a to $a + 5$ in the observed population, and P_{sa} denotes the proportion that currently married women aged a to $a + 5$ are of all currently married women aged 15–49 in a standard population, taken here as married women by age for all of Pakistan as determined from the 1973 HED Survey. The standard proportions are 0.0600 (15–19), 0.1368 (20–24), 0.1605 (25–29), 0.1649 (30–34), 0.1651 (35–39), 0.1586 (40–44), and 0.1541 (45–49).

If age were exaggerated by the same amount at each age, the age pattern of fertility (the graph of age-specific birth rates against age) would be shifted rightward by the same amount but remain unaltered in shape, and no spurious changes in age-specific birth rates would be observed as a result of age misreporting. But if age exaggeration increases with age, the pattern is quite different. Consider, for example, fertility in the age group 45–49. Age exaggeration among these women raises the estimated age-specific birth rate at ages 45–49 because women reported at these ages are actually somewhat younger than they say they are. If age exaggeration increases with age, then the own-children estimate of the birth rate in this age group is higher for the cohort of reported ages 60–64 at the time of the survey than for the cohort of reported ages 50–54. Of these two rates for ages 45–49, the former relates to a period ten years earlier than does the latter; therefore, the birth rate for ages 45–49 shows a spurious decline during the intervening ten years.

If age exaggeration is selective for women of high parity, the inflated level of and spurious decline in age-specific birth rates and marital birth rates at the older reproductive ages are even more pronounced; such selectivity is plausible, because educated guesses of age are probably heavily influenced by parity.

Further evidence in support of the age exaggeration hypothesis is provided by comparing own-children estimates of the age pattern of marital fertility in Table 5.4 with the age pattern of marital fertility of the Hutterites, an American religious sect that has the highest overall marital fertility on record. The sequence of Hutterite age-specific marital birth rates is 300 (15–19), 550 (20–24), 502 (25–29), 447 (30–34), 406 (35–39), 222 (40–44), and 61 (45–49), implying a standardized marital general fertility rate (see footnote to Table 5.4) of 359.

The comparison of Hutterite rates with the schedules of marital fertility in Table 5.4 shows Pakistan fertility exceeding Hutterite fertility at ages 15–19 for 1967–71 and at ages 45–49 for both 1962–66 and 1967–71, and falling short at intermediate ages. Marital fertility at ages 45–49 in Table 5.4 exceeds Hutterite fertility at the same ages by a factor of approximately 2. Such exceedingly high estimates of marital fertility at ages 45–49 are highly improbable, but they could occur if the true ages of older women are, on average, lower than reported ages.

It is instructive to look also at own-children estimates of age-specific birth rates above age 50. (Own-children estimates of births to women above age 50 were not distributed to women in the reproductive ages 15–49, because, on the assumption that age exaggeration is at work, adding births back in without also adding women with exaggerated ages back in would bias birth rates in an upward direction at the reproductive ages; women with exaggerated ages could not be added back in because of our inability to estimate reasonably accurately their number and distribution by age.) Own-children estimates of overall age-specific birth rates for 1970, with births corresponding to children of age 3 at the time of the survey, are 49 for ages 50–54 and 30 for ages 55–59. These rates, which are impossibly high, again suggest major age exaggeration.

It is possible, of course, that in the process of matching children to mothers, large numbers of children are mistakenly assigned to older women, thus accounting for inflated rates at the older ages. Some erroneous matches occur, for example, when children of dead mothers are adopted by older women. Since the relation-to-household-head classification, which is the principal basis for matching, does not contain a separate category for adopted children, adopted children are treated perforce as if they were biological children.

But it is unlikely that mismatches of this kind are numerous enough to account for the large effects observed. Adoption is rare in Pakistan. Orphaned children are more commonly absorbed into joint households, which constitute roughly half of all households. One common pattern is for children to live with their grandparents, either paternal or maternal. But it is then likely that children are coded as grandchildren of head, so that it is not possible for them to be erroneously matched to their grandmother; instead they are left as unmatched (non-own) and distributed by age group of women in the same proportions as own children are distributed by age group of women. Therefore, this pattern of caring for orphaned children cannot account for the high levels of and sharp declines in estimated age-specific fertility at the older reproductive ages.

Another common pattern is for children of a dead mother to be absorbed into the household of a sister or sister-in-law of the dead mother. Given the coding categories used in the HED survey, mismatching can occur in this situation, but only when a child's grandfather is the head of the household or when the child has actually been adopted; the potential for mismatching is limited, however, because the matching algorithm does not match more children to a woman than the number she says she has still living among those she has ever borne. Given that mortality increases with age, this sister or sister-in-law is at least as likely to be younger than the dead mother (were she still alive) as older. Once again, therefore, it seems highly unlikely that mismatch could account for the observed fertility levels and patterns of change at the older reproductive ages. Age exaggeration still provides the most likely explanation of these implausible levels and patterns of change.

What about the suspicious increase in marital fertility at the younger reproductive ages? Own-children estimates of age-specific marital fertility at the younger ages in Table 5.4 show an implausibly large rise. The rise is especially large, almost 24 percent, at ages 15–19, to levels substantially exceeding Hutterite fertility at the same ages. Again the explanation could involve age exaggeration. Age exaggeration at the younger reproductive ages reduces own-children estimates of age-specific marital birth rates at these ages because, in contrast to the situation with older women, the curve of age-specific marital fertility is rising instead of falling. If women are younger than they say they are, age-specific rates are underestimated. If age exaggeration increases with age for younger women, the own-children estimate of the birth rate at, say, ages 15–19 is lower for the cohort aged 25–29 at the time of the survey than for the cohort aged 20–24. Of these two rates for ages 15–19, the former relates to a period five years earlier than does the latter. Therefore, the birth rate for ages 15–19 shows a spurious rise during the intervening five years.

A difficulty with this line of reasoning is its implication that the estimates of fertility at ages 15–19 are underestimates, much as estimates of age-specific rates at the older ages are overestimates. Yet we have seen in Table 5.4 that own-children estimates of marital fertility at ages 15–19 during the period 1967–71 are unrealistically high, substantially exceeding Hutterite marital fertility at the same ages.

A possible explanation of this apparent contradiction is that age exaggeration is selectively concentrated among women of high parity. If parity-selective age exaggeration is especially prevalent among those of ages 15–19 at the time of the survey, then the ratio of children aged 2–6 to women in their late teens and early twenties at the time of the survey—from which, roughly speaking, the own-children estimate of the birth rate at ages 15–19 for 1967–71 is derived—could be too high instead of too low. There could also be some minimizing of the ages of unmarried women in order to improve their marriage chances; and to the extent that these women are removed from the denominators of the estimated age-specific birth rates, these birth rates would be inflated.

Another possible contributing factor is that some of the spreading and flattening of the age curve of fertility that is apparent in the comparison with Hutterite fertility may be due to random errors in age reporting, which would have the effect of increasing birth rates at both extremes of the reproductive age span and reducing them in between. Finally it should be noted that the estimate of Hutterite fertility at ages 15–19 is considerably less accurate than estimates at older ages; hence the base of comparison is considerably less certain at these ages.

In subsequent research the own-children method was also applied to household samples from the 1975 Pakistan Fertility Survey and the 1978–79 Population, Labor Force, and Migration (PLM) Survey, and to a subsample of the 1981 Census. Figure 5.10 compares trends in the TFR derived from these four sources (Retherford et al. 1985). For clarity, the comparisons are shown in three panels, with results from two successive censuses at a time compared. It is evident that the same distorted trend, starting from about the same level and ending at about the same level, is repeated from one census or survey to the next. The comparison suggests that in fact fertility was approximately constant, at a TFR of about 7, over the entire estimation period. The value of about 7 is consistent with the number of children ever born at women's ages 45–49 reported in the 1975 Pakistan Fertility Survey, which was 7.0. (The mean number of children ever born in the 1973 HED Survey is 15–20 percent lower. The discrepancy is almost surely due to omissions in the HED Survey, relating to failure to mention dead children and children no longer living in the household. The PFS data on children ever born, on the other hand, were derived from carefully collected birth histories.)

In Figure 5.10 the estimated TFR trend from each source indicates a spurious fertility decline during the first eight years or so immediately preceding the census or survey. Does this decline arise mainly from age misreporting or mainly from an undercount of young children? Although a definitive answer to this question cannot be given, the evidence does suggest that age misreporting plays a predominant role. For one thing, when the fertility estimates are aggregated, as described in Chapter 2, for the entire fifteen-year estimation period preceding each census or survey, the TFR for the entire period is close to 7. For example, the TFR derived in this way from the 1973 HED Survey is 6.9, in substantial agreement with the value of 7.0 children ever born for women of ages 45–49 as reported in the 1975 Pakistan Fertility Survey. If undercount were a serious problem, one would expect the own-children estimate of the TFR for the entire estimation period to fall noticeably below reported average number of children ever born.

A spurious decline in the TFR in the years immediately preceding a census or survey could be due mainly to age exaggeration from rounding of children's ages to the next higher age. For example, at age 0, corresponding to the first year before the census or survey, it is possible that many children of 11 months and perhaps younger ages as well are rounded to 1 year of age, resulting in a deficit of children reported at age 0 and a corresponding underestimate of fertility during the first year before the survey. At age 1, corresponding to the second year before the survey, substantial rounding to two years may occur not only at 23 months of age but also at 22 and 21 months and perhaps even younger ages as well. Thus the tendency to round upward from age 1 to age 2 may be greater than the tendency to round upward from age 0 to age 1, resulting in an overall deficit at age 1. Upward rounding that is substantially more pronounced for 1-year-olds than for 0-year-olds may explain the frequent and often spurious finding that cumulative fertility is lower in the second year before the survey than in the first year. This pattern occurs not only in Pakistan but also in some other countries, as we shall see in the next chapter. At ages 2, 3, . . . , 8, it is plausible that the rate at which upward rounding increases with age diminishes with age, so that estimated fertility increases as one moves backward in time. At ages beyond 8 (corresponding to nine or more years before the survey), heap-

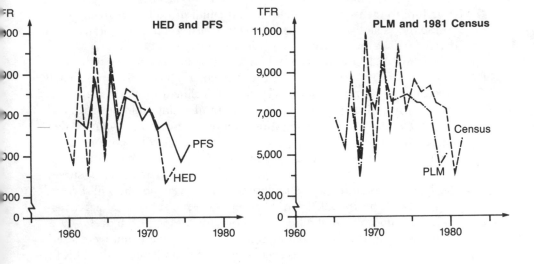

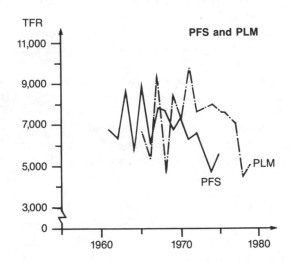

Figure 5.10. Own-children estimates of trends in the total fertility rate: Pakistan, various dates and sources

Source: Retherford et al. (1985:19).

Note: HED denotes Housing, Education, and Demographic Survey; PFS, Pakistan Fertility Survey; PLM, Population, Labor Force, and Migration Survey.

ing on ages 8, 10, and 12 predominates, resulting in sharp peaks in the TFR trend during the ninth, eleventh, and thirteenth years before the survey.

Figure 5.11 is similar to Figure 5.10, except that trends in age-specific birth rates (ASBRs) are graphed instead of TFRs. For brevity, only trends derived from the HED Survey and the 1981 Census are shown; the trends in ASBRs derived from the other two surveys show a rather similar pattern. The pattern of large fertility oscillations followed by a sharp fertility decline in the five years or so immediately preceding enumeration, with a slight upturn in the year just before enumeration, is found in every age group, and it again repeats from the first survey to the second, starting at approximately the same level and ending at approximately the same level. The indicated trends are clearly spurious. In reality, little systematic change in ASBRs occurred over the estimation period.

It is noteworthy that the trends in ASBRs derived from the HED Survey in Figure 5.11 do not show markedly different patterns of change over time at the younger and older ages. Instead, the pattern of trend distortion seems basically the same at all ages. This similarity seems inconsistent with the pattern of rising ASBRs at the younger ages (except 15–19) and falling ASBRs at the older ages, shown in Table 5.4, that was found in the earlier research based on the HED Survey. This inconsistency might stem from the way data were grouped in the earlier research: Children of ages 0 and 1 were ignored because it was thought that they were seriously undercounted, and fertility estimates were computed for two five-year time periods instead of for single calendar years, based on children aged 2–6 and 7–11 at the time of the survey. The time periods thus pertained to the third through seventh and eighth through eleventh years before the survey. Given the presence of major peaks and troughs in the estimated ASBR trends, as shown in Figure 5.11, it is possible that the manner in which the data were grouped could have affected the estimated trends. Indeed, it was found in the earlier research that grouping the data into four-year time periods yielded results quite different from those based on five-year time periods. But grouping the data into two five-year time periods yielded results quite similar to those based on two six-year time periods, suggesting that at this level of aggregation the choice of cutting points made little difference. It appears that aggregation over time periods as well as age exaggeration that increases with age may have introduced bias in the earlier results, but it is difficult to sort out the separate effects.

Like the Korean data discussed in the first part of this chapter, the Pakistani data illustrate the considerable analytical value of disaggregating

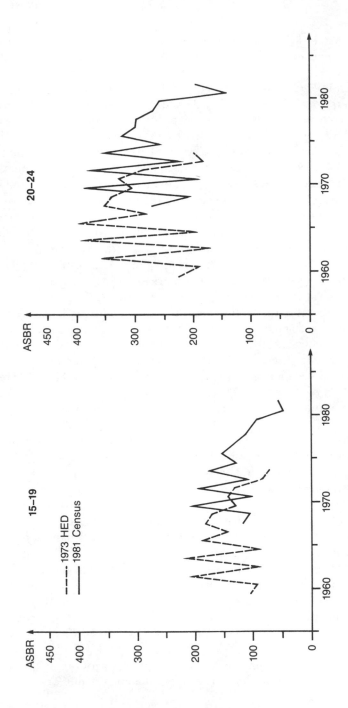

Figure 5.11. Own-children estimates of trends in age-specific birth rates derived from the 1973 Housing, Economic, and Demographic Survey and the 1981 Census: Pakistan, 1959–81

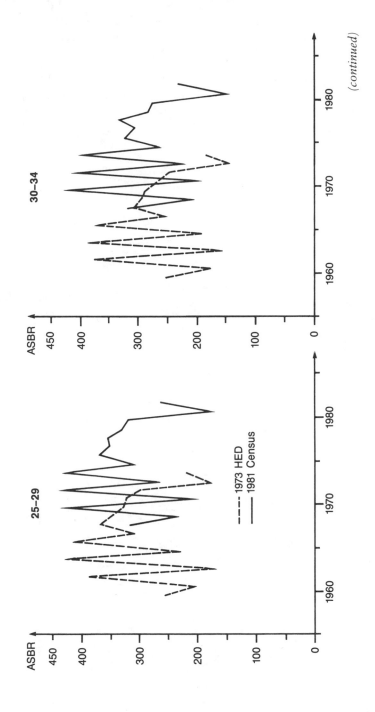

(continued)

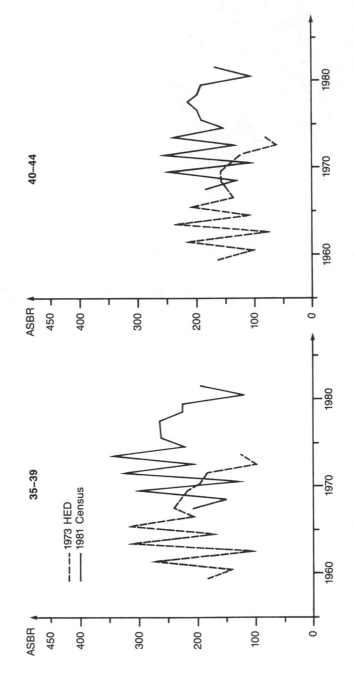

Figure 5.11. *(continued)*

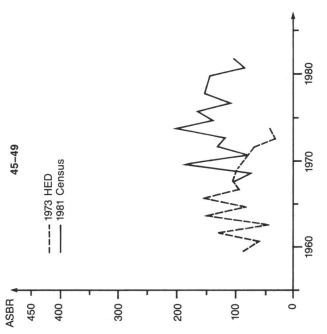

Sources: Retherford et al. (1985:20, 21) and unpublished tabulations.

fertility trends to show fertility estimates for single calendar years. In the case of Pakistan, this disaggregation reveals a typical pattern of distortion in the estimated trends that is largely hidden when the estimates are aggregated over five-year time periods. For both countries it is also evident that one more than doubles one's information by having at least two successive censuses or surveys instead of just one. The degree of agreement between overlapping trends is a valuable additional piece of information not available from either source separately. With results based on a single census or survey, one can never be quite sure whether a trend is spurious or real. But if the same suspected biases in estimated trends tend to be repeated in applications to successive censuses or surveys, comparisons of overlapping trends can yield reasonably firm conclusions about the degree of reality of the trend estimated from each source separately.

CHAPTER 6

Comparison of Fertility Trends Estimated Alternatively from Birth Histories and Own Children

It is of interest to compare fertility trends estimated alternatively from birth histories and own-children data because they are susceptible to many of the same kinds of estimation errors. Such comparisons have been made in an eight-country study based on data from the World Fertility Survey (Retherford and Alam 1985). This chapter presents principal findings from that study, and also from China's 1982 National Fertility Survey.

Findings from the World Fertility Survey

It is well known that both birth history analysis and own-children analysis frequently provide distorted estimates of fertility trends. The reasons for such distortions are imperfectly understood, however. In a widely cited article on estimating fertility trends from birth histories, Potter (1977) emphasized the role of event misplacement, which can lead to overestimating a decline in age-specific birth rates. He hypothesized that recent events are recorded fairly accurately but more distant events are misplaced toward the date of interview. The consequence is an artificial bunching of events five to ten years before the survey that results in a spuriously large estimated fertility decline for the ten years or so previous to the survey. Event misplacement tends to be associated with misreporting of children's ages. For example, an erroneous response that a child's age is, say, 11 years may be associated in a very direct way with a parallel erroneous response that the child's date of birth was eleven years previous to the survey.

The principal hypothesis examined here is that fertility trends estimated alternatively from birth histories and own-children data suffer from similar errors in the reporting of women's and children's ages and therefore should show a similar pattern of distortions from this source. It is

hypothesized additionally that the distortions are less pronounced in estimates of fertility trends derived from birth histories than in those derived
from own-children data. One expects this for several reasons. First, the
interviewer has more opportunity to notice and correct internal inconsistencies (for example, implausibly short birth intervals) when collecting
birth histories than when collecting own-children data. Second, questions on ages of children are usually more extensive and probing in the
birth histories than in the household surveys. Third, reporting by surro-
gates is absent in birth histories, where mothers invariably report for
themselves and their children, but frequent in household surveys, where
the household head often responds for the entire household. It should be
borne in mind that various methods of collecting birth histories were
employed in the World Fertility Survey (Jemai and Singh 1984), a fact
that affects the interpretation of findings presented here.

These hypotheses about similar sources of distortions in fertility estimates derived from birth histories and own-children data are tested on
World Fertility Survey (WFS) data from the Dominican Republic, Indonesia, Kenya, Republic of Korea, Nepal, Pakistan, Sri Lanka, and Syria.
Each of those country surveys covered a sample of either ever-married
women or, in the cases of the Dominican Republic and Kenya, both ever-
married and single women, from whom birth histories were collected.
The sample, called the individual sample, was embedded in a larger sample of complete households, called the household sample. In the study
reported here, the fertility trend is estimated alternatively from birth histories from the individual sample and from own-children data from the
household sample. The two estimated trends are then compared for each
of the eight countries.

Methodology. In the birth history approach, age-specific totals of
births to ever-married women are reconstructed from the birth histories
for each year previous to the survey. Person-years of exposure to risk for
ever-married women are similarly reconstructed. Except for the Dominican Republic and Kenya, where the individual sample included both
ever-married and single women, person-years at risk for all women,
regardless of their marital status, are estimated by dividing appropriate
age-specific categories of person-years at risk for ever-married women by
appropriate age-specific proportions ever married at the time of the survey. These proportions ever married are usually determined from the
WFS household samples; thus the birth history analysis is usually not
based entirely on the individual sample. In these computations, base calculations are done in century months, which are then aggregated to years
or groups of years as desired. The birth history approach ordinarily assumes that all births previous to the survey occurred to women who had

ever been married at the time of the survey and that none occurred to women still single (never married). It also assumes that women who died during the estimation period previous to the survey had, while they were alive, age-specific birth rates identical to those of women who survived. More detailed discussions of birth history analysis are found in numerous WFS publications (see, for example, Goldman, Coale, and Weinstein 1979).

In the present instance, the WFS computer program package, FERTRATE, was used to generate fertility estimates from birth histories. The time periods for which estimates were calculated were counted backward in twelve-month intervals starting from the time of the survey rather than from 1 January of the year of the survey, so that the estimates are comparable to those generated by the own-children method. The twelve-month intervals are labeled by the calendar year that encompasses most of the interval; for example, the period June 1978 to May 1979 would be labeled 1978, since more than half of the period fell in 1978.

The second approach to estimation utilizes the own-children method, which has already been described in earlier chapters. In this method, enumerated children are first matched to mothers within households, ordinarily on the basis of answers to questions on age, sex, marital status, number of children still living, and relation to head of household. WFS household surveys, however, contained a special code directly linking children to their mothers, so that matching was accomplished quite simply.

The own-children method requires life tables, from which reverse-survival ratios are computed. For the Dominican Republic, Republic of Korea, and Syria, constant mortality over time was assumed; and life tables were calculated by matching child mortality estimates, obtained by applying Brass's (1975) method to child survivorship data (numbers of children ever born and still living by age of mother) from the WFS survey itself, to the appropriate Coale–Demeny model West life table (Coale and Demeny 1966). For Indonesia we assumed changing mortality. Estimates of life expectancy for 1960 and 1978 were obtained from the United Nations 1976 and 1981 Demographic Yearbooks and were matched to Coale–Demeny model West life tables. These life tables were interpolated to single years of age and time by procedures described in Chapter 2 and Appendix A. A similar procedure was used for Kenya, except that the starting estimates for life expectancy were for 1969 and 1978. For Nepal we began with life expectancy estimates of 37.5 years for 1960 and 42.5 years for 1975 and then used the same procedure followed for Indonesia and Kenya. For Pakistan we assumed constant mortality and used the life table derived from the Population Growth Estimation (PGE) Survey of

1962–65 (Afzal 1974: 22). For Sri Lanka we assumed constant mortality and used published life tables for 1970–72 (Sri Lanka Department of Census and Statistics 1978).

As noted earlier, the own-children estimates are rather insensitive to errors in the mortality estimates because such errors cause only very small changes in reverse-survival ratios, which under modern mortality conditions are always rather close to 1. For the countries examined here, errors in the fertility estimates due to mortality estimation errors are much smaller than the errors stemming from age misporting. Moreover, the method of mortality estimation guarantees an absence of fluctuations over time in estimated mortality during the estimation period. Thus there is no danger whatever that year-to-year distortions in the estimated fertility trends, examined in the section of this chapter on results of the comparison, could be due to mortality estimation errors. Of course, our smoothing of mortality trends may have introduced some year-to-year distortions in the fertility estimates.

No adjustments for incorrect enumeration (age-selective sampling bias or age misreporting) were made, either in the birth history analysis or in the own-children analysis, since the effects of misenumeration, especially age misreporting, are of observational interest.

As mentioned, the own-children data include information on women up to 65 years of age. In the birth histories, however, only women below age 50 were queried. This means that, for the fifteen-year estimation period previous to the survey, annual estimates of complete age-specific fertility schedules covering the entire reproductive age range of 15–49 could be computed from the own-children data but not from the birth history data, which suffer from truncation as soon as one considers time periods previous to the survey. For example, if one wishes to compute age-specific birth rates for the fifth year previous to the survey from the birth histories, one is restricted to women aged 15–44 at that time instead of the full range of 15–49. For the full fifteen-year estimation period the range is restricted to ages 15–34. This has meant that the most desirable fertility measure, the total fertility rate, could not be used in comparing fertility trends estimated by the two methods. The cumulative fertility rate at exact age 35, CFR(35), calculated as five times the sum of age-specific birth rates for age groups 15–19 through 30–34, was used instead. Note the similarity to the total fertility rate, which is calculated in the same way but with a higher age cutoff.

The WFS data. The WFS samples were categorized into groups 1, 2, and 3.

In *Group 1,* which is the largest, the household and individual samples are the same, in that every woman in the individual sample belongs to a household in the household sample, and every eligible woman in every household of the household sample belongs to the individual sample (except for those few eligible women who were nonrespondents in the individual survey). Additionally, in the surveys in this group, field operations were carried out at approximately the same time and by the same field staff. Nepal, Pakistan, and Sri Lanka are in this group.

Given the almost simultaneous timing of the individual and household interviews for these countries, one might expect a close correspondence between the two samples in reported ages and birth dates. Preliminary tabulations indicated, however, that this was not always the case. A possible explanation of this lack of agreement hypothesizes the following sequence of events: Ages of all household members were first collected in the household interview. From the household schedule, ever-married women were identified. These women were subsequently questioned, and birth histories collected, in individual interviews. In the process of collecting birth histories, there was intensive questioning about birth intervals and dating of events, which resulted in some cases, by implication, in improved estimates of the respondent's or her children's ages. But these improved estimates are reflected in the household survey results only to the extent that someone, either in the field or in the office, took the trouble to go back to the household schedules and render the reports of women's and children's ages consistent with birth dates recorded in the birth histories. Apparently this was done much more completely in some countries than in others, and in some cases it may not have been done at all (Jemai and Singh 1984).

From published reports there is no way of knowing the extent to which consistency checking and resolving of discrepancies actually occurred, and this uncertainty results in an unknown degree of contamination that obscures the meaning of the comparisons to be made. The results for Pakistan and Nepal, however, suggest that little consistency checking was done, so that the comparisons seem unambiguous. In Sri Lanka, the third country in this group, age reporting is comparatively good, and there seems to be little consequent distortion in the trend estimates derived by either method.

The numbers of ever-married women in the individual sample and of persons in the household sample are 5,940 and 31,971 respectively for Nepal, 4,952 and 32,008 for Pakistan, and 6,810 and 47,914 for Sri Lanka.

In *Group 2* the individual sample is a subsample of the household sample, the latter generally covering three or four times as many households as the former. The two surveys were carried out at approximately the same time and by the same field staff, so that contamination is not excluded, but it is clearly less serious than in the countries in Group 1 because it can affect only the minority of mothers who were selected for the individual survey. In the present study three countries fall into Group 2: the Dominican Republic, Republic of Korea, and Syria. In the Dominican Republic the women in the individual sample were sampled directly from a list of all the eligible women in the household sample (i.e., there was no process of subsampling households). In Korea and Syria the individual sample consists of all eligible women in a subsample of the households of the household sample.

The numbers of ever-married women in the individual sample and of persons in the household sample are 3,115 and 59,493 for the Dominican Republic, 5,430 and 104,892 for Korea, and 4,487 and 97,310 for Syria.

In *Group 3* the individual and household schedules (the household schedule was very short) were administered in the same interview, so that this case represents the most extreme form of contamination of all three groups. Indonesia and Kenya fall into this category. In the case of Indonesia, however, this difficulty can be largely circumvented because the WFS household survey, known as SUPAS III, was embedded in a much larger survey known as SUPAS II. Thus fertility trends can be estimated by the own-children method from SUPAS II as well as from SUPAS III, both of which we examine here. Because of the large sample size of SUPAS II, the own-children fertility estimates derived from it are relatively free of contamination. No such remedy for contamination was available for Kenya, and the results for Kenya are therefore less instructive than those for the other countries.

The numbers of ever-married women in the individual sample and of persons in the household sample are 9,155 and 50,994 for Indonesia and 8,100 and 46,101 for Kenya. The SUPAS II sample, of which the WFS household sample SUPAS III is a subsample, contains 281,168 persons.

Results of the comparison. Findings are presented in the order of the three groups discussed above. Trends in cumulative fertility rates to age 35, CFR(35), estimated alternatively from birth histories and own-children data, are summarized in Figure 6.1. (Similar graphs for ASBRs are presented in Retherford and Alam 1985.)

Results for Nepal are presented in Panel A of Figure 6.1. The CFR estimates derived by the own-children method (Panel A of Figure 6.1) show a pattern that has been found to be fairly typical for countries of continental South Asia, namely large oscillations during the period ten to fourteen years before the survey and a substantial fertility decline during the eight years or so immediately preceding the survey. Usually the estimates show a fertility upturn in the year just preceding the survey, and this is also evident for Nepal. We have already observed this pattern for Pakistan in chapters 4 and 5.

The large oscillations during the period ten to fourteen years before the survey reflect severe heaping on children's ages of 10 and 12, corresponding to births in the eleventh and thirteenth years before the survey. The comparatively low fertility during the first five years or so immediately preceding the survey may be due mainly to age exaggeration from rounding of children's ages to the next higher age. This pattern resembles that found for Pakistan, as discussed earlier in Chapter 5.

The parallel CFR trend based on birth histories for Nepal (Panel A of Figure 6.1) bears only a slight resemblance to that based on own-children data. On the whole the estimates based on birth histories show little change over time, indicating an absence of fertility decline, and the comparatively minor year-to-year fluctuations do not parallel very closely those derived from own-children data. The results seem either to contradict the hypothesis that fertility trends based alternatively on birth histories and own-children data reflect the same age-reporting errors, or to suggest that the survey takers made exceptional efforts, through probing, to achieve a degree of consistency in the reporting of the timing of birth events in the birth histories that left few traces of age misreporting.

The impressively smooth results from birth histories may have something to do with the Takeshita method of collecting birth histories. This method, which was used in Nepal but not in most other WFS countries, makes special efforts to obtain accurate age data (Jemai and Singh 1984). The smooth results from the birth histories may also be related to extensive imputation of dates of events collected in the birth histories (Chidambaram and Sathar 1984). But imputation cannot be the main reason for the smooth trend derived from the Nepalese birth histories because, as we shall see, this trend is much less smooth in Pakistan, where imputation was just as extensive as in Nepal. If age misreporting is the principal cause of whatever year-to-year distortions remain in the fertility trend estimates for Nepal, then it is apparent that little or no effort was made to render birth dates in the individual sample and ages in the household sample consistent with each other.

The pattern of own-children estimates for Pakistan (Panel B of Figure 6.1) is quite similar to that for Nepal, with pronounced fertility fluctuations early in the estimation period, substantial fertility decline subsequently, and a small upturn in the year immediately preceding the survey; but age misreporting seems more severe, as indicated by more jagged patterns. Again major peaks in the fertility trend occur in the eleventh and

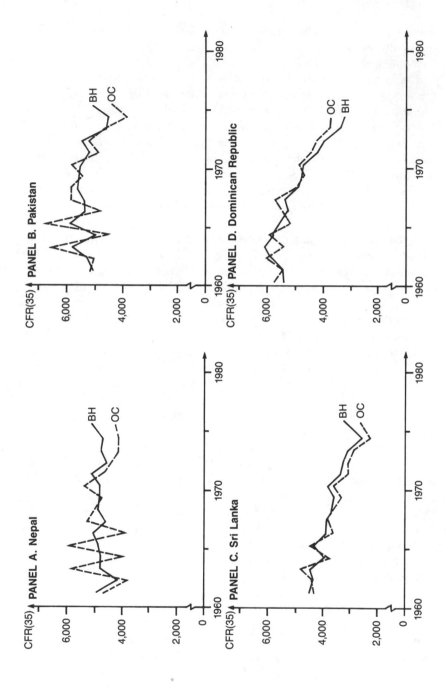

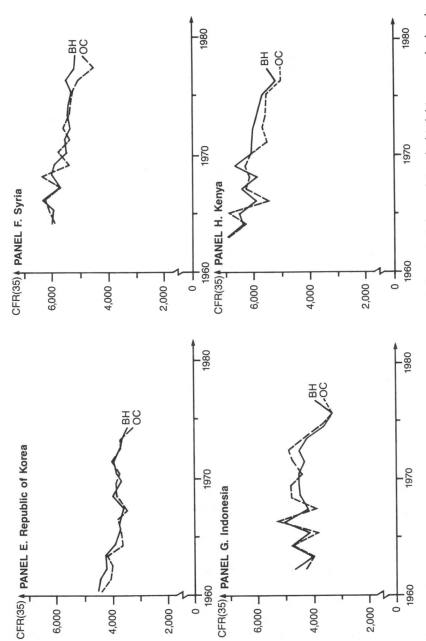

Figure 6.1. Trends in cumulative fertility rates, CFR (35), estimated alternatively by applying the birth history method and the own-children method to the World Fertility Survey: Various countries and periods

Source: Retherford and Alam (1985).

Note: BH denotes birth histories; OC, own-children data.

thirteenth years previous to the survey, corresponding to heaping on ages 10 and 12. Consonant with our initial hypothesis, the fertility trends estimated by the own-children method are considerably more jagged than those estimated from birth histories, and they show a similar pattern of year-to-year fluctuations. Peaks and troughs in the estimated trends derived by the two methods coincide rather closely. Thus the Pakistan data tend to support the hypothesis that fertility trends estimated alternatively from birth histories and own-children data suffer from similar biases due to similar age-reporting errors in both data sets.

Results for the third country in Group 1, Sri Lanka (Panel C of Figure 6.1), show annual fluctuations in the trends estimated alternatively from birth histories and own children that tend to rise and fall together, and this pattern again supports the hypothesis that the two trends are similarly biased by age-reporting errors. There tend to be peaks in the sixth, ninth, eleventh, and thirteenth years before the survey, corresponding to heaping on ages 5, 8, 10, and 12. The heaping is minor, however, in keeping with the comparatively accurate age reporting that is known to characterize Sri Lanka (Ratnayake, Retherford, and Sivasubramaniam 1984).

In Sri Lanka as well as in Nepal and Pakistan there tends to be a small fertility upturn in the year immediately preceding the survey. Overall, the recurring pattern of fertility peaks corresponding to children's ages 0, 8, 10, and 12 strongly suggests that the observed peaks and troughs in the fertility trends are due primarily to age misreporting and do not reflect real annual fluctuations in fertility. (Note, however, that sampling errors for single-year rates in WFS surveys are large; see Little 1982.)

Next are the Group 2 countries, for which, it will be recalled, the individual sample is embedded in a considerably larger household sample. For the Dominican Republic (Panel D of Figure 6.1) the trends estimated alternatively from birth histories and own-children data coincide reasonably closely, except for the five years immediately preceding the survey, in which fertility is seen to decline more steeply for the birth history estimates than for the own-children estimates. In the estimates derived by the own-children method there appears to be some heaping on ages 4, 7, 10, and 12, corresponding to local peaks in the fertility trend in the fifth, eighth, eleventh, and thirteenth years before the survey. (Nepal, Pakistan, and Sri Lanka also showed heaping on ages 10 and 12.) The trend estimated from birth histories also shows local peaks in the fifth and eighth years before the survey, but not in the eleventh or thirteenth year; instead, it peaks in the twelveth year before the survey. Age reporting errors, described in a previous WFS study (Guzman 1980), are implicated in these patterns, despite their inconsistencies.

Similar graphs of ASBRs (not shown) indicate that the relatively steep fertility decline estimated from birth histories during the five years immediately preceding the Dominican Republic survey is due mainly to discrepancies between the birth history and own-children trends at maternal ages 15–19, much less so to discrepancies at ages 20–24, and hardly at all to discrepancies at ages 25–29 and 30–34. Possibly age-specific proportions ever married from the household sample were underestimated at the younger reproductive ages, resulting in an excessive deflation of birth rates for ever-married women at these ages when these latter rates were effectively multiplied through by age-specific proportions ever married to estimate birth rates for women of all marital statuses combined. Such an error would result in fertility underestimates derived from the birth histories. Given well-known difficulties in assessing the extent of consensual unions (which are especially prevalent at the younger reproductive ages) as opposed to formal unions in many Caribbean countries, this seems a plausible source of error.

The relatively smooth estimated fertility decline since 1965 in the Dominican Republic suggests that age-reporting problems are not severe and that the downward trend in fertility is real. This impression is reinforced by information on contraceptive use rates, which the WFS found to be substantial: Fully 97 percent of eligible women knew of at least one modern contraceptive method, and 26 percent were using one (Hobcraft and Rodriguez 1982).

Results for the Republic of Korea, the second country in Group 2 (Panel E of Figure 6.1) show a CFR decline in the 1960s, a temporary rise in the late 1960s and early 1970s, and a resumption of the decline in the 1970s. The temporary fertility resurgence in the late 1960s and early 1970s has also been observed in fertility trends estimated from other sources (see, for example, Retherford, Cho, and Kim 1983) and seems to be real. The resurgence is most noticeable for age-specific birth rates at ages 20–24 and 25–29, which suggests that the resurgence was due to shifts in the timing of births due to unprecedented prosperity in the late 1960s and early 1970s, rather than to a temporary reversal of the downward trend of completed fertility. Age reporting is known to be very accurate in Korea, and there is no indication in Figure 6.1 that the small annual fluctuations in the two sets of fertility trends based alternatively on birth histories and own-children data reflect common patterns of age misreporting, which is largely absent.

Results for Syria, the third country in Group 2 (Panel F of Figure 6.1) show quite good agreement between the CFR trends estimated alternatively from birth histories and own-children data during all but the most recent three years of the estimation period, in which the trend from the own-children data drops below the trend from birth histories. The peaks and troughs of the fertility trends estimated alternatively from birth histories and own-children data do not coincide very consistently.

As mentioned, the Group 3 countries, Indonesia and Kenya, have the greatest degree of mutual contamination between birth histories and own-children data, since both the individual and the household schedules were administered during the same interview. As anticipated, (Panel G of Figure 6.1) the peaks and troughs of the fertility trends estimated for Indonesia alternatively from birth histories and own-children data coincide rather well, and, as hypothesized, the oscillations over time tend to be more pronounced for the own-children estimates than for the birth history estimates. The pattern of peaks and troughs resembles that for Nepal and Pakistan; that is, the peaks correspond to children's ages 10 and 12, and there is an apparent fertility decline in the five years or so immediately preceding the survey, with a slight upturn in the year just before the survey.

As mentioned earlier, an additional comparison is possible in the case of Indonesia, because the WFS household sample, known as SUPAS III, was embedded in a much larger household survey known as SUPAS II. Figure 6.2 compares own-children estimates of trends in the TFR, covering the entire reproductive age range of 15–49, derived from SUPAS II and SUPAS III. It shows that the pattern of peaks and troughs due to age misreporting is quite similar in the two surveys but tends to be somewhat more pronounced in the WFS SUPAS III than in SUPAS II. This pattern of discrepancies again tends to support the hypothesis that the collection of birth histories results in a good deal of checking for internal consistency that ultimately provides better, or at least more consistent, estimates of women's and children's ages and the timing of birth events. The age–event chart used as an aid in collecting birth histories in Indonesia, as in Nepal, probably contributed to the quality of the age data obtained (Jemai and Singh 1984; Supraptilah 1982).

For the last country in Group 3, Kenya, again the fertility trends indicate severe contamination between the individual and household samples (Panel H of Figure 6.1). As in the case of Indonesia, the CFR(35) trends estimated alternatively from birth histories and own children coincide rather well, although the trend derived from own-children data tends to be somewhat lower than the trend derived from birth histories in the first seven years or so immediately preceding the survey. Again there is some indication of heaping on ages 8, 10, and 12, corresponding to fertility peaks in the ninth, eleventh, and thirteenth years before the survey; a subsequent decline in fertility; and a slight upturn in the year just preceding the survey. As in the other countries, year-to-year fluctuations tend to

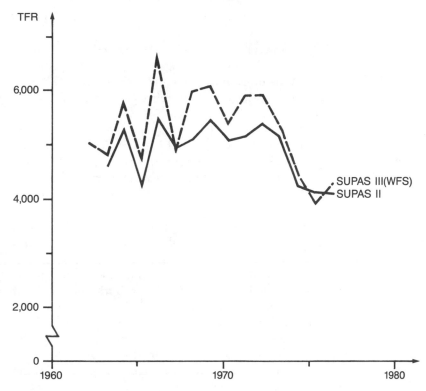

Figure 6.2. Own-children estimates of trends in total fertility rates derived from SUPAS II and SUPAS III: Indonesia, 1962–76

Source: Retherford and Alam (1985).

be larger in the own-children estimates than in the birth history estimates. Again this suggests that even though the household and individual schedules were administered in the same interview, birth dates and ages were not always rendered consistent in the two schedules. The data for Kenya tend also to support the original hypothesis that distortions in fertility trends estimated alternatively from birth histories and own-children data reflect similar age-reporting errors.

Discussion. From the ages of surviving children matched to a woman in the own-children procedure, one can infer birth dates, yielding a partial birth history that omits births of children who later died or moved out of the household before being enumerated in the survey. In effect, the own-children adjustments for mortality and unmatched children compensate for these omissions. Thus, as noted in Chapter 1, the own-children method may be regarded as fertility estimation from incomplete maternity histories.

Given this similarity between the own-children method and the birth history method, our initial hypothesis, that fertility trends estimated alternatively from birth histories and own children tend to suffer from similar errors in age reporting that should be reflected in roughly coinciding peaks and troughs in the estimated year-to-year fertility trends, is supported fairly strongly by the results for Pakistan, Sri Lanka, Indonesia, and Kenya, but only weakly or not at all by the results for Nepal, the Dominican Republic, Korea, and Syria. Our further hypothesis, that distortions due to age misreporting should be more pronounced in the trend derived from own-children data than in the trend derived from birth histories, which offer more opportunity to detect and correct internal inconsistencies during interviews of respondents, is supported by the results for Nepal, Pakistan, the Dominican Republic, Syria, Indonesia, and Kenya, but weakly or not at all by the reports for Korea and Sri Lanka. In the case of Nepal, it is possible that an extraordinary effort was made to obtain birth histories with a smooth sequence of birth intervals, and that this effort left little trace of the typical South Asian pattern of age misreporting so evident in the own-children estimates. This may have been due partly to use of an age–event chart of the type recommended by Takeshita for the collection of birth histories. In Korea age reporting is known to be quite accurate, and the impact of age misreporting on the estimated fertility trends seems to be minimal. In most cases the agreement between the fertility estimates derived alternatively from own-children data and birth histories is impressive.

None of the countries examined shows much indication of a bunching of births in the birth histories in the vicinity of five to ten years before the survey; fertility ten to fourteen years before the survey tends to be about as high or higher than fertility five to ten years before the survey. Moreover, in at least one case, Pakistan, fertility during the five years immediately preceding the survey seems implausibly low, probably owing to a pattern of age exaggeration stemming from upward rounding of children's ages. Additional evidence in support of this hypothesis, based on overlapping fertility trends estimated from successive censuses or surveys, has already been examined in Chapter 5. This mechanism probably operates in Indonesia as well, although independent evidence indicating a rapid rise in contraceptive use suggests that part of the indicated fertility decline in Indonesia is real. On the whole, Potter's hypothesis about misplacement of events, which assumes bunching of births five to ten years before the survey and accurate reporting of births during the first five years or so immediately preceding the survey, does not receive much support from these data. This finding reinforces previous work by Blacker and Brass (1979), who also found evidence that recent birth dates obtained from birth histories tend to be pushed backward from, rather than toward, the survey date.

Findings from China's 1982 National Fertility Survey

The own-children method has also been applied to China's 1982 National Fertility Survey, which is known to have been extraordinarily accurate (Cho, Han, and Li 1985). The sample size for this survey was very large, amounting to 1,017,574 persons. The sampling fraction was approximately 1/1,000. Like the WFS, this survey used both a household questionnaire and an individual questionnaire. The individual questionnaire was administered to sample women 15–67 years of age, instead of the usual range of 15–49 (Wang and Xiao 1984).

The survey included a simple household questionnaire that was originally intended to aid in the identification of eligible women, to whom the individual questionnaire was administered. The own-children method was later applied to the household data to obtain estimates of fertility for years between 1963 and 1982. The data were of sufficient quality that estimates could be computed for a period up to twenty years before the survey instead of the usual fifteen years before the survey. Life tables for reverse survival were obtained by matching age-specific death rates estimated by Wang (1984) to an appropriate Coale–Demeny model North life table.

The fertility estimates derived alternatively from birth histories and own-children data in the 1982 survey are compared in Figure 6.3. In this case it is possible to examine total fertility rates instead of cumulative fertility rates to age 35 because the birth histories were asked of women aged 15–67 instead of 15–49, thereby eliminating the truncation problem discussed earlier in connection with the WFS surveys. The annual estimates derived by the own-children method overlap calendar years, whereas the annual estimates derived from the birth histories correspond strictly to calendar years (January to December). In Figure 6.3 the estimates derived from birth histories incorporate a one-half year adjustment to facilitate comparison with the estimates derived by the own-children method.

The agreement between the two trends is excellent, especially for the first fifteen years before the survey. The still good agreement for the period sixteen to twenty years before the census is noteworthy because,

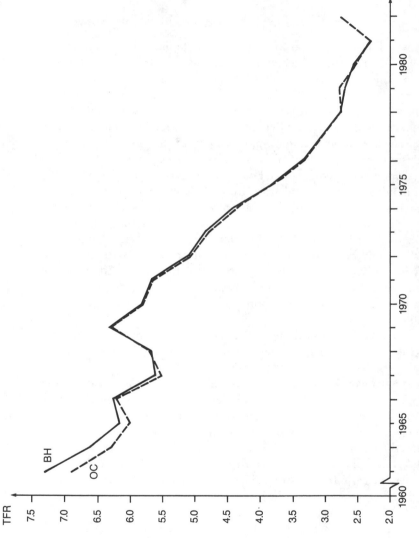

Figure 6.3. Trends in total fertility rates estimated alternatively by applying the birth history method and the own-children method to the 1982 National Fertility Survey: China, 1963–82

Source: Unpublished tabulations.

in the own-children estimates, births for this early period are derived from children aged 15–19, a substantial proportion of whom no longer live in the parental household and therefore cannot be matched to their mothers. Peaks and troughs in the estimated trends coincide rather closely. The deviation between the two trends during the period 1966–81 never exceeds 1.5 percent, except for 1979, when the deviation is slightly larger.

CHAPTER 7

Step-by-Step Procedure with Illustrative Results for Thailand

This chapter presents details of the basic own-children estimation procedure, with emphasis on results from each of three major stages of computer programs.

The three-stage procedure

The computational procedure for the own-children method is organized in three major stages. First, children below age 15 are matched, where possible, to their mothers. Second, from the matched data file obtained in the first stage, women are tabulated by age, own children are tabulated by child's age and mother's age, and non-own children are tabulated by child's age. Third, annual age-specific birth rates and derived fertility measures are computed from the tabulations from the second stage. The results of each stage may be saved on computer tape for use in the next stage or in further analyses. Background tabulations from a study by Arnold, Pejarananda, and Choe (1986) are used here as a source of illustrative results from stages 2 and 3. These results, presented later in this chapter, are derived from an application of the own-children method to the 1980 Census of Thailand.

Of the three stages, the first is the most data-dependent, in that the stage-1 computer program requires the most modification before it can be adapted from one data set to another. Modifications are necessary to conform to the format of the questionnaire data and to the specification of information used for matching, particularly the coding categories of relationship to head of household. The programs for the other two stages are more standardized. Examples of computer programs are given in Appendix C.

Stage 1: matching

Matching of children to mothers is accomplished by a computerized matching algorithm. The following conditions must be met for matching to be accomplished: (1) the census or survey must be of households; (2) there must be a separate record for each person in the household; (3) the records for individual persons must be grouped by household; (4) separate households must be identified either by a unique household number or by a housing record preceding the records for persons in the household; and (5) each person's record must include data on age, sex, and relationship to head of household. If each woman's record contains information on marital status, this information may be employed to restrict matches to ever-married women. If each woman's record contains information on number of children ever born or number of children surviving, this information is employed so that no more children are matched to a woman than the number she says are still living among those she has ever borne. If the reports on children ever born and still living are classified by sex of child, this information is also employed so that no more boys are matched to a woman than the number of boys she says are still living among those she has ever borne, and likewise for girls.

Because many children begin to live away from their mothers starting at about age 15, matching is usually limited to children younger than 15. This age limit determines the time period for which fertility rates are to be estimated. If the limit is 15, it is possible to estimate fertility rates for each year up to and including the fifteenth year before the census. In the following discussion, age 14 (corresponding to births in the fifteenth year before the census) is assumed to be the upper age limit of children for matching purposes.

The matching algorithm begins by scanning a household, saving information on all women in the age range 15–65 as potential mothers and all children below age 15 as potential own children. Normally, never-married women are not considered to be potential mothers, but this restriction can be relaxed if illegitimate births are common. For each potential mother, considered in the order listed in the household schedule, a search is made of all children in the household who have not yet been matched to a woman. For each of these children, the child's relationship code is compared with the woman's relationship code. When the two codes are compatible with a mother–child match, the ages of the woman and child are compared. If the age difference falls in the range 15–49, the child is matched to that woman.

For a particular woman, the search for her own children stops when the number of children matched to her reaches the reported number of her living children or after all the unmatched children in the household have been scanned. The children below age 15 who are not matched to a woman by the end of the household scan are considered non-own children.

The matching procedure yields a new data file with two record types. The first record type is a woman record. A woman record is created for each woman between the ages of 15 and 65 inclusive, containing the characteristics of the woman and the age and sex of each of her own children below age 15, if any. The second record type is a non-own-children record. A non-own-children record is created for each household with non-own children. The record contains the age and sex of each un-matched child below age 15 in the household.

The following hypothetical example illustrates the procedure. Consider a household of eight persons with the following selected information:

Person number	Relationship to head of household	Sex	Marital status	Age	Number of living children
1	head	M	M	55	—
2	wife	F	M	53	4
3	son	M	M	30	—
4	daughter-in-law	F	M	28	2
5	daughter	F	D	21	0
6	son	M	N	12	—
7	granddaughter	F	N	5	—
8	grandson	M	N	2	—

The marital status code M denotes currently married, D denotes divorced, and N denotes never married. In this census the information on number of living children was asked of women of ages 15 and older only. For this household the matching algorithm creates the following list of potential mothers:

Person number	Relationship	Marital status	Age	Number of living children
2	wife	M	53	4
4	daughter-in-law	M	28	2
5	daughter	D	21	0

It then goes on to create the following list of potential own children:

Person number	Relationship	Sex	Age
6	son	M	12
7	granddaughter	F	5
8	grandson	M	2

For the first potential mother listed, the relationship code is wife. Therefore, among the potential own children only the first child with person number 6 has a relationship code that is consistent with being her child. The age difference is 53 − 12 = 41, which is within the acceptable range. The woman can have up to four children matched to her. To start with, the number matched to her is zero. Thus, the child with person number 6 is determined to be the woman's own child. Similarly, children with person numbers 7 and 8 are matched to the woman with person number 4. No children are matched to the woman with person number 5 because she has no living children. In any case, no children are left to be matched to her. In this household there are no non-own children. Three records corresponding to three potential mothers are generated as follows:

Person number	Information from woman's record					Own-children					
						Sex	Age	Sex	Age	Sex	Age
2	wife	F	M	53	4	M	12	—	—	—	—
4	daughter-in-law	F	M	28	2	F	5	M	2	—	—
5	daughter	F	D	21	0	—	—	—	—	—	—

In actual applications, additional information such as geographical area and socioeconomic characteristics is included in the woman records, and age and sex of each child are included in the non-own children records. Each output record has a flag indicating whether the record is a woman record or a non-own-children record.

If mother's person number is collected for each child below age 15, matching is much simpler. In our example the household is then processed on the basis of the following information:

Person number	Sex	Marital status	Age	Mother's person number
1	M	M	55	—
2	F	M	53	—
3	M	M	30	—
4	F	M	28	—
5	F	D	21	—
6	M	N	12	2
7	F	N	5	4
8	M	N	2	4

The list of potential mothers is then

Person number	Marital status	Age
2	M	53
4	M	28
5	D	21

And the list of potential own-children is

Person number	Sex	Age	Mother's person number
6	M	12	2
7	F	5	4
8	M	2	4

The first woman on the list of potential mothers has person number 2. The matching algorithm matches children with mother's person number 2 to her. In our example one child is so matched. The second woman has person number 4, and all children with mother's person number 4 are matched to her. In this case two children are matched. No children are matched to the third woman because no children have mother's person number 5.

The procedure based on mother's person number (MPN matching) is simpler and usually results in more accurate matching than the procedure based on relation to household head (RHH matching). To modify our example, suppose that the woman with person number 4 in the above example has one child living away from home, and that the woman with person number 5 is the mother of the child with person number 8. Then the household list will look the same as before, except that the number of living children for person number 5 is changed to 1. For this household, RHH matching produces the same result as before, which is now incorrect. The difficulty is the ambiguity of the relationship of grandson, who can be either daughter's son or daughter-in-law's son. In contrast, MPN matching gives correct results in this modified example.

Most applications of the own-children method use RHH matching because mother's person number is not usually available. It is sometimes asked for in populations where complex households with many potential mothers are common, to improve the accuracy of matching and thereby to facilitate application of the own-children method.

Stage 2: basic tabulation

The second stage of the procedure tabulates data from the matched records from the first stage. The basic tabulation shows numbers of women by age, numbers of own children by child's age and mother's age, and numbers of non-own children by child's age. Table 7.1 is an example of the basic table, based on an application of the own-children method to the 1980 Census of Thailand. Results are shown only for the whole kingdom. A similar table is produced for each geographic subdivision and each category of each socioeconomic variable considered.

Stage 2 also has an option for calculating and printing numbers of children ever born per woman and children surviving per woman by age in five-year age groups. A tabulation of these child survivorship data is again produced for whatever geographic subdivisions and socioeconomic variables are specified. In the case of Thailand, the child survivorship data were tabulated independently by the National Statistical Office and are not shown.

Stage 3: computation of fertility estimates

As a preliminary to stage 3, the child survivorship data just described were used to obtain estimates of infant mortality trends by Feeney's method (Feeney 1980). Infant mortality rate (IMR) estimates for 1974–76 so derived were compared with corresponding estimates from Thailand's 1974–76 Survey of Population Change (SPC). It was found that the estimates derived by Feeney's method were lower than those from the SPC. The ratio of the SPC estimate of the IMR to the estimate of the IMR derived by Feeney's method for 1974–76 was used as an adjustment factor to adjust upward the estimates of the IMRs derived by Feeney's method, regardless of the year to which they pertained. The adjusted IMR for each calendar year was then matched to the appropriate level of the Coale–Demeny North model life table family. In this way a complete abridged life table was obtained for each calendar year during the fifteen-

Table 7.1. Women by age, children by own age and mother's age, and

Women's age	No. of women	0	1	2	3	4	5
15	6,071	34	15	7	0	0	0
16	5,716	93	38	15	8	0	0
17	5,665	212	95	40	16	8	0
18	5,401	337	184	86	42	16	10
19	5,103	465	297	176	94	39	18
20	5,264	639	455	324	217	102	50
21	5,016	636	502	402	301	165	87
22	5,217	729	609	534	459	301	189
23	4,768	756	669	628	583	442	334
24	4,231	714	639	627	625	521	441
25	3,971	661	642	633	659	588	542
26	3,641	595	570	609	621	590	574
27	3,628	578	551	591	654	622	631
28	3,253	483	476	515	573	571	598
29	3,308	468	475	509	579	585	649
30	3,184	414	414	460	540	554	598
31	2,655	332	334	376	432	465	514
32	2,639	305	314	354	416	439	502
33	2,345	250	256	285	358	367	432
34	2,197	218	226	266	315	334	391
35	2,292	207	219	257	306	334	387
36	1,970	167	173	203	251	268	320
37	2,210	177	183	222	256	289	335
38	2,026	152	160	187	228	243	303
39	2,393	160	180	207	259	281	327
40	2,186	123	136	168	205	229	273
41	1,981	110	120	151	184	201	248
42	1,928	89	100	131	161	186	222
43	1,863	68	82	106	143	156	201
44	1,740	51	66	89	115	145	174
45	1,817	35	49	70	97	123	160
46	1,669	25	40	51	80	97	134
47	1,665	21	28	40	59	80	109
48	1,457	13	17	27	40	54	77
49	1,470	11	13	19	28	41	64
50	1,416	9	11	14	20	28	44
51	1,350	10	9	12	15	22	30
52	1,130	6	8	9	12	15	18
53	1,137	7	7	7	7	10	13
54	996	4	5	7	7	8	8
55	914	0	5	6	6	7	9
56	919	0	0	4	5	6	6
57	809	0	0	0	4	4	6
58	788	0	0	0	0	4	5
59	776	0	0	0	0	0	5
60	707	0	0	0	0	0	0
61	642	0	0	0	0	0	0
62	609	0	0	0	0	0	0
63	657	0	0	0	0	0	0
64	524	0	0	0	0	0	0
65	501	0	0	0	0	0	0
Non-own children		773	783	794	839	813	877

non-own children by age: Thailand, 1980

Children's Age								
6	7	8	9	10	11	12	13	14
0	0	0	0	0	0	0	0	0
0	0	0	0	0	0	0	0	0
0	0	0	0	0	0	0	0	0
0	0	0	0	0	0	0	0	0
11	0	0	0	0	0	0	0	0
28	19	0	0	0	0	0	0	0
39	20	13	0	0	0	0	0	0
95	46	22	15	0	0	0	0	0
192	109	53	29	22	0	0	0	0
310	207	112	55	34	25	0	0	0
415	312	198	105	63	39	29	0	0
482	394	273	169	92	53	33	24	0
571	503	405	279	182	102	51	30	21
564	532	451	354	252	149	89	44	24
619	625	570	480	381	274	171	95	47
625	607	601	547	472	375	280	171	100
534	561	555	528	476	421	320	220	126
526	555	583	560	538	493	421	315	206
457	487	525	538	514	502	443	368	271
419	448	496	512	511	495	476	395	326
424	460	499	533	532	538	520	459	409
349	379	420	449	456	480	475	418	391
383	414	463	497	506	534	531	516	470
328	359	408	440	452	482	497	463	468
382	416	466	522	527	574	597	561	565
307	337	395	413	461	474	509	496	500
285	306	358	391	410	444	463	448	473
241	281	323	352	376	415	437	426	445
226	270	300	331	346	384	413	400	423
198	229	277	299	319	348	373	362	393
185	226	258	294	316	344	372	362	385
162	199	234	259	284	311	339	326	356
140	175	213	241	261	300	319	314	340
107	128	167	195	211	244	271	261	280
86	118	151	174	205	230	252	260	280
59	87	120	138	165	197	218	226	249
46	68	98	123	144	179	213	213	236
27	42	62	78	99	128	153	158	178
17	26	40	53	79	106	125	140	168
13	16	22	34	49	78	90	105	132
10	13	18	24	36	50	68	77	101
6	9	13	17	24	34	49	65	82
6	9	9	11	15	23	33	44	58
6	8	8	10	11	17	23	30	45
5	5	6	7	8	12	14	22	32
3	4	5	5	8	8	10	12	18
0	5	5	5	6	8	7	11	12
0	0	4	5	5	6	6	7	11
0	0	0	5	4	5	5	7	6
0	0	0	0	3	4	4	5	5
0	0	0	0	0	0	0	0	0
938	1,034	1,094	1,133	1,192	1,269	1,372	1,419	1,556

year estimation period preceding the 1980 Census. These abridged life tables were interpolated to single years of age by procedures described in Chapter 2 and Appendix A. The mortality estimates were part of the input to stage 3.

Further input to stage 3 included a set of correction factors for undercount and misenumeration (the factors U_x^c and U_a^w in equations [2.7] to [2.11] in Chapter 2), a set of age-specific proportions married in five-year age groups (for use in computing age-specific marital birth rates for the year before the census), and a standard age distribution in five-year age groups for ages 15–49 (for use in computing age-standardized general fertility rates). The age-specific proportions married were calculated from the census itself, and the standard age distribution was chosen in this case as a Coale–Demeny Model North stable population with a life expectancy at birth for males and females of 60 years (Coale and Demeny 1966). Of course the output from stage 2 was also part of the input for stage 3.

The first results printed by the stage-3 program summarize that part of the input for stage 3 that does not come directly from stage 2. Table 7.2 presents the input correction factors U_x^c and U_a^w, the derivation of which need not concern us here. Table 7.3 presents the proportions married and the standard age distribution. (The results in these two tables are not well labeled in the printed output and have been reformatted here for the reader's convenience.)

The next table printed out by stage 3 is the interpolated single-year life tables for each of the fifteen years immediately preceding the census, by sex. To conserve space, only the person-years (L_x) column of the life table is printed out, since that column is used to construct reverse-survival ratios. In addition, life expectancy at birth is printed out as a summary index of mortality. For brevity, since the computer-printed table is lengthy, Table 7.4 presents only the estimates of life expectancy at birth, by sex, for each of the fifteen years during the estimation period preceding the 1980 Census.

The first major output table from stage 3 is a period–cohort birth matrix and a period–cohort woman matrix, for use in computing period–cohort birth rates. Estimates of these quantities for Thailand are shown in Tables 7.5 and 7.6. Recall from Chapter 2, Figure 2.1, that period–cohort births and women (actually woman-years of exposure) for parallelograms in the Lexis plane are the quantities that flow most naturally from the process of reverse survival. The estimates of period–cohort births and women in Tables 7.5 and 7.6 refer to parallelograms of the type AB and CD in Figure 2.1. Note that Tables 7.5 and 7.6 are tabulated by survey age rather than age at the time the births actually occurred. This means that one can follow real cohorts (defined by survey age)

Table 7.2. Age-specific correction factors, U_x^c and U_a^w, used in applying the own-children method to the 1980 Census: Thailand

Age	Correction factor	Age	Correction factor
Children		Women *(continued)*	
0	1.085	32	1.000
1	1.085	33	1.000
2	1.085	34	1.000
3	1.085	35	1.000
4	1.085	36	1.000
5	1.085	37	1.000
6	1.085	38	1.000
7	1.085	39	1.000
8	1.085	40	1.000
9	1.085	41	1.000
10	1.085	42	1.000
11	1.085	43	1.000
12	1.085	44	1.000
13	1.085	45	1.000
14	1.085	46	1.000
		47	1.000
Women		48	1.000
15	1.000	49	1.000
16	1.000	50	1.000
17	1.000	51	1.000
18	1.000	52	1.000
19	1.000	53	1.000
20	1.000	54	1.000
21	1.000	55	1.000
22	1.000	56	1.000
23	1.000	57	1.000
24	1.000	58	1.000
25	1.000	59	1.000
26	1.000	60	1.000
27	1.000	61	1.000
28	1.000	62	1.000
29	1.000	63	1.000
30	1.000	64	1.000
31	1.000	65	1.000

Note: For explanation of U_x^c and U_a^w see equations (2.7) to (2.11) in Chapter 2.

backward in time by reading rightward across rows. A table of period–cohort age-specific birth rates could be produced by term-by-term division of Table 7.5 by Table 7.6. The program does not do this because the single-year rates are not usually of interest. One typically aggregates Tables 7.5 and 7.6 into age groups and time periods with a hand calculator, as desired, before dividing them term-by-term to obtain birth rates. The mode of aggregation is not standard and depends on the application.

Table 7.3. Age-specific proportions married from the 1980 Census and standard age distribution for calculation of age-standardized fertility measures in stage 3 of the own-children fertility estimation procedure: Thailand

Age group	Proportions currently married	Standard population
15–19	.1559	437,800
20–24	.5295	431,463
25–29	.7432	423,798
30–34	.8201	415,125
35–39	.8438	405,299
40–44	.8325	394,022
45–49	.7989	380,623

Note: The standard age distribution is taken from a Coale-Demeny model West stationary population with a life expectancy for females of 60 years (Coale and Demeny 1966).

Table 7.4. Estimates of life expectancy, by sex, for each of the fifteen years preceding the 1980 Census: Thailand

Year	Female	Male
1979	65.05	61.37
1978	64.55	60.87
1977	64.05	60.36
1976	63.55	59.86
1975	63.04	59.36
1974	62.54	58.86
1973	62.04	58.36
1972	61.54	57.86
1971	61.04	57.36
1970	60.54	56.87
1969	60.04	56.37
1968	59.54	55.88
1967	59.03	55.38
1966	58.53	54.89
1965	58.03	54.40

Tables 7.7 and 7.8 are similar to Tables 7.5 and 7.6 except that they pertain to age–period, or central, births and women instead of period–cohort births and women. The central births and women pertain to squares in the Lexis plane, again as illustrated by Figure 2.1 in Chapter 2. They are calculated using the averaging procedure described in Chapter 2. In this case the tabulations are by woman's age in previous years rather than her age at the time of the census or survey. Table 7.9, which presents age-specific central birth rates by single years of age for single calendar years, is obtained by term-by-term division of Table 7.7 by Table 7.8.

Although birth rates for single calendar years often are of interest, it is rare that birth rates by single years of age are of interest. Therefore, another basic tabulation routinely printed out is central births and woman-years of exposure, with ages grouped into standard five-year age categories, as shown in Tables 7.10 and 7.11. These tables are obtained directly from Tables 7.7 and 7.8 by aggregation.

Tables 7.12 and 7.13, which provide estimates of central age-specific birth rates and summary measures for five-year age groups, are the main output tables of interest. The first part of Table 7.12 presents age-specific birth rates for single calendar years, obtained by term-by-term division of Table 7.10 by Table 7.11. Also presented are two estimates of the total fertility rate, one pertaining to ages 15–44 and the other to ages 15–49. (Note that TFRs in Table 7.12 are not identical to those in Table 7.9, although the basic data are exactly the same. Discrepancies are introduced because age distributions are not rectangular within five-year age groups.) Four estimates of the general fertility rate (GFR) are given, corresponding to the two age ranges 15–44 and 15–49 and to whether the actual age distribution or the standard age distribution is used. The general fertility rate is calculated as

$$\text{GFR} = (\Sigma_a P_a^f F_a)/(\Sigma_a P_a^f), \tag{7.1}$$

where P_a^f denotes the number of women aged a to $a + 5$, F_a denotes the central age-specific birth rate for ages a to $a + 5$, and the summations range over either 15–44 or 15–49. If the GFR is standardized, standard instead of observed values of P_a^f are used.

Table 7.13 presents results for aggregated time periods, derived from Tables 7.10 and 7.11. As explained in Chapter 2, numerators and denominators of rates are first aggregated into age groups and time periods by the program before they are divided to get rates. In Table 7.13 the program allows as many as ten time groupings, which are specified by the user.

Table 7.5. Period–cohort births, by women's age, estimated by applying the own-

		Number of years					
Women's age	No. of women	<1 1979	1 1978	2 1977	3 1976	4 1975	5 1974
15	6,071	41	18	8	0	0	0
16	5,716	113	48	19	11	0	0
17	5,665	258	119	51	21	10	0
18	5,401	410	231	109	54	21	13
19	5,103	567	372	224	120	51	24
20	5,264	778	570	411	278	132	65
21	5,016	775	628	510	385	213	113
22	5,217	888	763	677	587	388	246
23	4,768	921	837	796	745	570	435
24	4,231	870	799	794	799	673	574
25	3,971	804	804	803	843	759	705
26	3,641	724	714	773	794	761	747
27	3,628	704	689	750	837	803	822
28	3,253	588	596	653	733	737	778
29	3,308	570	594	645	740	754	845
30	3,184	504	518	584	690	714	778
31	2,655	405	418	476	552	599	669
32	2,639	371	393	449	532	566	653
33	2,345	305	321	362	458	474	562
34	2,197	266	282	337	403	430	509
35	2,292	252	274	325	392	431	503
36	1,970	204	216	258	321	345	417
37	2,210	216	229	281	327	372	436
38	2,026	185	200	237	292	314	394
39	2,393	195	225	262	331	363	426
40	2,186	149	170	213	262	295	355
41	1,982	134	150	192	236	260	323
42	1,928	109	125	166	205	240	290
43	1,863	82	103	134	183	201	262
44	1,740	62	83	113	147	187	226
45	1,817	43	61	89	124	159	208
46	1,669	30	50	65	102	125	175
47	1,665	26	35	50	75	104	142
48	1,457	16	22	34	51	70	100
49	1,470	13	16	24	36	52	83
50	1,416	11	14	18	25	36	57
51	1,351	13	12	15	19	28	39
52	1,130	8	10	11	15	19	24
53	1,137	8	8	8	9	12	17
54	996	5	7	9	9	10	11
55	914	0	6	7	7	9	11
56	919	0	0	5	6	7	8
57	809	0	0	0	5	5	8
58	788	0	0	0	0	5	7
59	776	0	0	0	0	0	6
60	707	0	0	0	0	0	0
61	642	0	0	0	0	0	0
62	609	0	0	0	0	0	0
63	657	0	0	0	0	0	0
64	524	0	0	0	0	0	0
Total	125,312	12,621	11,730	11,947	12,764	12,306	13,066
Non-own factor		1.0746	1.0836	1.0843	1.0840	1.0853	1.0874

preceding the census and actual year

6 1973	7 1972	8 1971	9 1970	10 1969	11 1968	12 1967	13 1966	14 1965
0	0	0	0	0	0	0	0	0
0	0	0	0	0	0	0	0	0
0	0	0	0	0	0	0	0	0
0	0	0	0	0	0	0	0	0
15	0	0	0	0	0	0	0	0
37	26	0	0	0	0	0	0	0
51	27	18	0	0	0	0	0	0
126	61	30	21	0	0	0	0	0
253	146	72	40	31	0	0	0	0
409	278	151	76	47	35	0	0	0
547	417	267	144	87	55	42	0	0
636	527	370	231	128	74	47	35	0
754	674	548	381	252	143	73	44	32
745	713	609	484	350	209	127	64	36
818	836	770	656	528	385	245	138	70
825	812	813	748	655	527	401	250	149
705	751	750	723	660	592	458	321	189
694	743	788	766	747	692	602	461	308
603	652	710	735	712	705	633	539	405
553	600	671	700	709	695	681	578	489
559	616	675	729	738	756	743	672	613
460	508	569	614	632	675	679	611	585
505	554	626	679	702	750	759	756	705
432	481	552	602	627	676	711	678	701
504	556	631	714	731	806	854	821	846
405	451	535	564	639	666	728	725	749
376	410	485	535	568	624	662	656	709
318	376	437	481	522	583	624	623	666
298	362	405	453	479	540	591	585	634
262	306	375	409	442	489	534	529	589
245	303	349	403	438	484	533	529	577
213	267	316	354	394	436	485	477	533
184	234	288	329	362	422	456	459	509
141	171	225	266	293	343	388	382	420
113	157	205	238	284	324	360	380	419
78	117	162	188	229	277	312	331	374
60	91	133	168	200	251	305	311	354
36	56	83	107	138	180	218	231	267
22	35	54	72	110	149	179	205	251
17	22	30	47	68	110	129	154	198
13	18	24	33	50	71	97	113	152
8	12	17	23	33	48	69	95	123
8	12	13	15	21	33	47	64	87
8	11	11	14	15	24	33	44	68
6	7	8	10	11	16	20	32	48
4	5	7	7	11	11	14	17	27
0	6	6	7	8	11	10	16	17
0	0	5	6	7	8	9	10	17
0	0	0	7	6	7	8	11	9
0	0	0	0	4	5	5	7	8
13,046	13,406	13,792	13,778	13,667	13,887	13,871	12,954	12,935
1.0949	1.1033	1.1073	1.1125	1.1209	1.1283	1.1414	1.1603	1.1803

Table 7.6. Period–cohort woman-years of exposure, by women's age, estimated

							Number of years
Women's age	<1 1979	1 1978	2 1977	3 1976	4 1975	5 1974	6 1973
15	6,071	0	0	0	0	0	0
16	5,716	5,726	0	0	0	0	0
17	5,665	5,675	5,686	0	0	0	0
18	5,401	5,411	5,422	5,432	0	0	0
19	5,103	5,113	5,123	5,134	5,144	0	0
20	5,264	5,276	5,287	5,298	5,309	5,320	0
21	5,016	5,028	5,039	5,050	5,061	5,072	5,083
22	5,217	5,229	5,242	5,254	5,266	5,278	5,290
23	4,768	4,780	4,792	4,804	4,816	4,827	4,838
24	4,231	4,242	4,253	4,264	4,275	4,286	4,296
25	3,971	3,981	3,992	4,003	4,013	4,024	4,034
26	3,641	3,651	3,661	3,671	3,681	3,691	3,701
27	3,628	3,638	3,648	3,659	3,669	3,680	3,690
28	3,253	3,263	3,272	3,282	3,291	3,301	3,311
29	3,308	3,318	3,328	3,338	3,348	3,358	3,369
30	3,184	3,194	3,204	3,214	3,224	3,234	3,244
31	2,655	2,663	2,671	2,680	2,688	2,697	2,706
32	2,639	2,647	2,656	2,665	2,673	2,682	2,691
33	2,345	2,353	2,361	2,369	2,377	2,385	2,393
34	2,197	2,204	2,212	2,219	2,227	2,235	2,242
35	2,292	2,300	2,308	2,316	2,324	2,332	2,341
36	1,970	1,977	1,984	1,991	1,998	2,006	2,013
37	2,210	2,218	2,226	2,234	2,243	2,251	2,259
38	2,026	2,034	2,042	2,049	2,057	2,065	2,073
39	2,393	2,402	2,412	2,421	2,431	2,440	2,450
40	2,186	2,196	2,205	2,214	2,223	2,231	2,241
41	1,981	1,990	1,999	2,007	2,016	2,024	2,033
42	1,928	1,937	1,946	1,955	1,963	1,972	1,980
43	1,863	1,872	1,881	1,890	1,899	1,907	1,916
44	1,740	1,749	1,757	1,766	1,774	1,783	1,791
45	1,817	1,826	1,836	1,845	1,854	1,864	1,873
46	1,669	1,677	1,686	1,695	1,704	1,713	1,722
47	1,665	1,674	1,683	1,692	1,701	1,710	1,719
48	1,457	1,465	1,474	1,482	1,490	1,498	1,507
49	1,470	1,479	1,487	1,496	1,504	1,513	1,522
50	1,416	1,426	1,435	1,443	1,452	1,460	1,469
51	1,350	1,360	1,369	1,378	1,387	1,395	1,404
52	1,130	1,139	1,147	1,155	1,163	1,170	1,177
53	1,137	1,147	1,156	1,164	1,173	1,181	1,188
54	996	1,005	1,013	1,021	1,029	1,037	1,044
55	914	923	931	939	946	954	961
56	919	927	936	944	953	961	968
57	809	817	825	833	841	848	856
58	788	797	805	813	821	829	836
59	776	786	795	803	811	819	827
60	707	716	725	734	742	749	757
61	642	652	660	669	677	684	691
62	609	619	628	636	645	652	660
63	657	668	679	689	699	708	717
64	524	534	543	552	561	569	577
Total	125,312	119,702	114,420	109,161	104,142	99,395	94,457

by applying the own-children method to the 1980 Census: Thailand

preceding the census and actual year

7 1972	8 1971	9 1970	10 1969	11 1968	12 1967	13 1966	14 1965	15 1964
0	0	0	0	0	0	0	0	0
0	0	0	0	0	0	0	0	0
0	0	0	0	0	0	0	0	0
0	0	0	0	0	0	0	0	0
0	0	0	0	0	0	0	0	0
0	0	0	0	0	0	0	0	0
0	0	0	0	0	0	0	0	0
5,301	0	0	0	0	0	0	0	0
4,849	4,861	0	0	0	0	0	0	0
4,307	4,317	4,327	0	0	0	0	0	0
4,045	4,055	4,065	4,075	0	0	0	0	0
3,711	3,721	3,730	3,740	3,749	0	0	0	0
3,700	3,711	3,720	3,730	3,740	3,750	0	0	0
3,320	3,330	3,339	3,349	3,358	3,367	3,376	0	0
3,379	3,389	3,399	3,409	3,419	3,428	3,438	3,448	0
3,254	3,264	3,274	3,284	3,294	3,304	3,313	3,323	3,332
2,714	2,723	2,732	2,741	2,749	2,758	2,766	2,774	2,783
2,700	2,709	2,718	2,727	2,736	2,745	2,753	2,762	2,770
2,401	2,409	2,417	2,426	2,434	2,442	2,450	2,458	2,466
2,250	2,258	2,266	2,274	2,282	2,290	2,298	2,306	2,313
2,349	2,357	2,366	2,375	2,383	2,392	2,400	2,409	2,417
2,020	2,028	2,036	2,043	2,051	2,058	2,066	2,074	2,081
2,268	2,276	2,285	2,294	2,303	2,311	2,320	2,329	2,338
2,081	2,089	2,097	2,106	2,114	2,122	2,131	2,139	2,147
2,460	2,469	2,479	2,489	2,499	2,509	2,520	2,530	2,540
2,250	2,259	2,268	2,278	2,287	2,296	2,306	2,316	2,325
2,041	2,050	2,058	2,067	2,076	2,085	2,094	2,103	2,112
1,989	1,997	2,006	2,015	2,023	2,032	2,041	2,050	2,059
1,924	1,933	1,941	1,950	1,959	1,968	1,976	1,985	1,994
1,799	1,808	1,816	1,824	1,833	1,841	1,850	1,858	1,867
1,882	1,891	1,900	1,908	1,917	1,927	1,936	1,945	1,954
1,730	1,739	1,747	1,756	1,764	1,773	1,782	1,790	1,799
1,729	1,738	1,746	1,755	1,764	1,773	1,782	1,791	1,799
1,515	1,523	1,531	1,539	1,547	1,555	1,563	1,571	1,579
1,530	1,539	1,547	1,556	1,564	1,573	1,581	1,589	1,598
1,477	1,486	1,495	1,503	1,512	1,520	1,528	1,537	1,545
1,412	1,420	1,429	1,437	1,446	1,454	1,462	1,471	1,479
1,185	1,192	1,199	1,207	1,214	1,221	1,228	1,236	1,243
1,196	1,203	1,211	1,219	1,226	1,234	1,241	1,249	1,256
1,051	1,057	1,064	1,071	1,078	1,085	1,092	1,099	1,106
968	974	981	987	994	1,000	1,007	1,013	1,020
976	983	990	996	1,003	1,010	1,016	1,023	1,030
863	869	876	882	888	894	900	906	913
844	851	857	864	870	876	882	889	895
835	842	849	856	863	869	875	882	888
764	772	779	785	792	798	804	810	816
698	705	712	719	725	731	737	743	748
667	674	681	687	694	700	706	712	717
725	733	741	749	756	763	770	777	783
584	591	597	604	610	616	622	628	634
89,742	84,794	80,273	76,274	72,515	69,071	65,614	62,522	59,347

Table 7.7. Age–period (central) births, by women's age, estimated by applying

| | | | | | | Number of years | |
Women's age	<1 1979	1 1978	2 1977	3 1976	4 1975	5 1974	6 1973
15	77	83	80	87	91	89	88
16	185	175	166	199	173	179	189
17	334	301	317	332	301	340	331
18	488	471	460	486	479	505	478
19	672	599	593	666	621	640	592
20	776	695	736	772	716	726	695
21	831	800	795	821	760	784	749
22	904	818	799	819	782	800	781
23	895	802	788	816	770	811	821
24	837	759	761	785	746	811	765
25	764	701	702	737	734	724	699
26	714	643	649	715	657	661	649
27	646	595	615	621	583	608	578
28	579	556	530	542	520	535	556
29	537	468	463	495	452	506	509
30	455	406	406	431	431	460	483
31	388	357	350	398	388	426	469
32	338	301	331	356	359	415	468
33	285	278	292	324	343	410	454
34	259	245	270	309	338	391	390
35	228	223	259	311	329	339	347
36	210	215	250	297	278	306	308
37	200	213	238	249	250	276	280
38	190	197	202	221	220	244	253
39	172	160	179	194	194	217	229
40	142	138	150	165	173	191	199
41	121	114	123	136	142	158	163
42	96	93	101	113	114	121	127
43	72	72	77	89	87	92	95
44	53	55	57	63	61	70	69
45	37	42	42	44	44	48	48
46	28	28	29	31	32	32	29
47	21	19	21	22	24	20	20
48	14	15	16	17	16	14	15
49	12	13	13	12	11	11	11
50	12	11	10	9	10	10	8
51	10	9	9	8	8	8	8
52	8	7	8	7	6	7	7
53	7	6	6	6	5	6	5
54	3	3	3	3	3	3	2
55	0	0	0	0	0	0	0
56	0	0	0	0	0	0	0
57	0	0	0	0	0	0	0
58	0	0	0	0	0	0	0
59	0	0	0	0	0	0	0
60	0	0	0	0	0	0	0
61	0	0	0	0	0	0	0
62	0	0	0	0	0	0	0
63	0	0	0	0	0	0	0

preceding the census and actual year

7 1972	8 1971	9 1970	10 1969	11 1968	12 1967	13 1966	14 1965
104	111	110	107	109	100	101	110
212	209	187	190	176	186	194	169
347	318	306	301	297	323	285	248
472	459	432	439	456	429	391	357
601	579	570	592	559	530	500	447
693	690	702	657	642	617	559	551
774	791	735	703	699	657	625	599
824	781	745	729	700	712	641	645
781	769	751	711	726	711	683	703
747	749	718	723	715	719	717	774
697	690	714	685	712	735	749	798
626	673	671	667	713	782	773	729
608	622	646	664	741	791	691	688
562	597	640	679	736	695	639	650
531	589	658	685	645	643	604	611
518	592	639	604	603	607	557	583
519	583	550	545	561	562	529	555
504	510	508	501	514	533	503	521
430	461	467	461	486	509	468	464
393	421	431	440	460	471	420	419
369	390	406	416	429	422	381	396
334	362	378	378	382	374	356	364
305	333	341	327	333	336	321	311
285	302	298	288	301	308	271	259
250	257	252	256	264	262	218	224
202	215	213	214	215	198	179	175
164	183	178	169	164	154	134	138
137	147	138	124	130	113	104	105
104	108	90	89	90	83	80	77
74	69	59	59	59	58	54	58
46	42	40	42	40	40	38	38
29	27	28	27	28	26	24	22
20	20	19	18	20	17	16	17
15	15	14	13	14	12	13	13
12	12	12	11	11	9	11	9
11	10	9	10	9	8	9	9
9	7	7	8	8	7	7	7
6	6	7	7	6	6	6	6
5	6	7	5	5	5	5	5
3	3	3	3	3	3	3	3
0	0	0	0	0	0	0	0
0	0	0	0	0	0	0	0
0	0	0	0	0	0	0	0
0	0	0	0	0	0	0	0
0	0	0	0	0	0	0	0
0	0	0	0	0	0	0	0
0	0	0	0	0	0	0	0
0	0	0	0	0	0	0	0

Table 7.8. Central woman-years of exposure, by women's age, estimated by

						Number of years	
Women's age	<1 1979	1 1978	2 1977	3 1976	4 1975	5 1974	6 1973
15	5,899	5,706	5,559	5,288	5,232	5,201	5,192
16	5,696	5,548	5,278	5,221	5,191	5,181	5,070
17	5,538	5,267	5,211	5,180	5,170	5,058	4,572
18	5,257	5,200	5,168	5,158	5,047	4,562	4,170
19	5,189	5,157	5,147	5,035	4,551	4,160	3,873
20	5,146	5,135	5,023	4,540	4,150	3,863	3,701
21	5,123	5,011	4,528	4,139	3,852	3,691	3,505
22	4,998	4,517	4,128	3,842	3,680	3,495	3,345
23	4,505	4,117	3,831	3,670	3,485	3,335	3,311
24	4,106	3,821	3,660	3,475	3,325	3,301	2,979
25	3,811	3,649	3,465	3,315	3,291	2,970	2,703
26	3,639	3,455	3,305	3,281	2,960	2,694	2,546
27	3,445	3,295	3,271	2,951	2,685	2,537	2,321
28	3,286	3,261	2,942	2,676	2,529	2,313	2,296
29	3,251	2,933	2,668	2,521	2,306	2,288	2,181
30	2,924	2,659	2,512	2,298	2,280	2,173	2,140
31	2,651	2,504	2,290	2,272	2,165	2,133	2,170
32	2,496	2,282	2,264	2,157	2,125	2,162	2,266
33	2,275	2,256	2,150	2,117	2,154	2,258	2,350
34	2,248	2,142	2,109	2,146	2,249	2,340	2,141
35	2,135	2,102	2,138	2,240	2,331	2,132	2,011
36	2,094	2,130	2,232	2,322	2,123	2,002	1,952
37	2,122	2,223	2,313	2,115	1,994	1,944	1,858
38	2,214	2,303	2,106	1,985	1,935	1,849	1,836
39	2,294	2,097	1,977	1,927	1,841	1,828	1,802
40	2,088	1,968	1,918	1,832	1,819	1,793	1,725
41	1,959	1,909	1,823	1,810	1,784	1,716	1,617
42	1,900	1,815	1,801	1,774	1,707	1,608	1,518
43	1,806	1,792	1,765	1,698	1,600	1,510	1,500
44	1,783	1,756	1,689	1,591	1,501	1,491	1,440
45	1,747	1,680	1,582	1,493	1,482	1,432	1,294
46	1,671	1,574	1,485	1,474	1,424	1,286	1,187
47	1,565	1,476	1,465	1,415	1,279	1,179	1,120
48	1,468	1,457	1,407	1,271	1,172	1,112	1,006
49	1,448	1,398	1,262	1,164	1,105	999	968
50	1,388	1,254	1,156	1,097	992	961	915
51	1,245	1,147	1,089	984	954	908	850
52	1,138	1,080	976	946	901	842	836
53	1,071	968	938	893	835	828	796
54	959	929	885	827	820	788	728
55	921	876	819	812	780	720	679
56	868	811	804	772	713	672	692
57	803	796	764	705	664	685	650
58	787	755	697	657	676	642	0
59	746	688	648	668	634	0	0
60	679	640	659	625	0	0	0
61	630	649	616	0	0	0	0
62	639	606	0	0	0	0	0
63	595	0	0	0	0	0	0

preceding the census and actual year

7 1972	8 1971	9 1970	10 1969	11 1968	12 1967	13 1966	14 1965
5,081	4,594	4,201	3,912	3,750	3,563	3,412	3,390
4,583	4,191	3,902	3,740	3,554	3,403	3,380	3,053
4,181	3,893	3,730	3,544	3,393	3,371	3,044	2,772
3,883	3,721	3,535	3,384	3,361	3,035	2,764	2,614
3,711	3,525	3,374	3,352	3,026	2,756	2,606	2,386
3,515	3,365	3,342	3,017	2,747	2,597	2,378	2,362
3,355	3,332	3,007	2,738	2,589	2,370	2,353	2,245
3,321	2,998	2,729	2,580	2,362	2,345	2,237	2,206
2,988	2,720	2,572	2,354	2,337	2,229	2,198	2,238
2,712	2,563	2,346	2,329	2,221	2,189	2,230	2,339
2,554	2,338	2,320	2,213	2,181	2,221	2,330	2,427
2,329	2,312	2,205	2,173	2,212	2,321	2,418	2,214
2,304	2,196	2,165	2,204	2,312	2,408	2,204	2,081
2,188	2,157	2,195	2,302	2,398	2,195	2,072	2,022
2,148	2,187	2,293	2,388	2,186	2,063	2,013	1,926
2,179	2,284	2,378	2,177	2,054	2,004	1,917	1,906
2,275	2,369	2,168	2,045	1,996	1,909	1,897	1,872
2,359	2,159	2,037	1,987	1,900	1,888	1,863	1,795
2,150	2,028	1,978	1,891	1,880	1,854	1,786	1,685
2,019	1,969	1,883	1,871	1,845	1,777	1,676	1,584
1,961	1,874	1,862	1,836	1,769	1,668	1,576	1,567
1,866	1,854	1,828	1,760	1,660	1,568	1,559	1,508
1,845	1,819	1,751	1,651	1,560	1,550	1,499	1,357
1,810	1,743	1,643	1,552	1,542	1,491	1,349	1,246
1,734	1,634	1,544	1,534	1,483	1,341	1,239	1,177
1,626	1,535	1,525	1,475	1,334	1,231	1,170	1,059
1,527	1,517	1,466	1,326	1,224	1,163	1,053	1,022
1,508	1,458	1,318	1,216	1,156	1,046	1,015	968
1,449	1,310	1,209	1,148	1,039	1,008	961	901
1,302	1,201	1,141	1,032	1,002	955	894	888
1,194	1,134	1,026	995	948	888	882	849
1,127	1,019	989	942	882	876	843	779
1,013	982	936	876	870	837	773	730
975	929	870	863	830	767	724	748
922	863	857	824	761	719	741	705
857	850	817	755	713	735	699	0
843	810	749	706	729	693	0	0
803	742	700	722	686	0	0	0
735	693	715	679	0	0	0	0
686	707	672	0	0	0	0	0
700	665	0	0	0	0	0	0
658	0	0	0	0	0	0	0
0	0	0	0	0	0	0	0
0	0	0	0	0	0	0	0
0	0	0	0	0	0	0	0
0	0	0	0	0	0	0	0
0	0	0	0	0	0	0	0
0	0	0	0	0	0	0	0
0	0	0	0	0	0	0	0

Table 7.9. Central age-specific birth rates, by women's age, estimated by apply-

Women's age				Number of years			
	<1 1979	1 1978	2 1977	3 1976	4 1975	5 1974	6 1973
15	13.1	14.6	14.4	16.5	17.5	17.2	17.0
16	32.6	31.5	31.5	38.1	33.3	34.6	37.3
17	60.3	57.2	60.9	64.0	58.2	67.3	72.3
18	92.9	90.5	89.0	94.3	95.0	110.6	114.6
19	129.5	116.1	115.2	132.3	136.6	153.8	152.8
20	150.8	135.4	146.6	170.1	172.5	187.9	187.7
21	162.2	159.6	175.6	198.3	197.2	212.5	213.8
22	180.9	181.1	193.5	213.1	212.4	228.9	233.6
23	198.7	194.7	205.6	222.2	220.9	243.3	248.0
24	203.8	198.6	208.0	225.8	224.2	245.8	256.8
25	200.6	192.2	202.5	222.2	223.1	243.7	258.8
26	196.2	186.0	196.4	218.0	221.9	245.5	254.9
27	187.5	180.6	187.9	210.5	217.1	239.5	249.0
28	176.2	170.5	180.2	202.5	205.7	231.4	242.1
29	165.3	159.6	173.5	196.4	196.1	221.2	233.7
30	155.5	152.6	161.5	187.5	188.9	211.7	225.5
31	146.3	142.6	152.7	175.0	179.3	199.9	216.1
32	135.4	132.1	146.4	165.1	168.9	191.9	206.6
33	125.4	123.2	135.7	153.1	159.3	181.6	193.4
34	115.0	114.3	127.8	144.2	150.4	166.9	182.4
35	106.6	106.0	121.3	139.0	141.2	159.1	172.6
36	100.1	100.9	111.9	127.8	130.7	153.0	157.7
37	94.4	95.6	102.7	117.8	125.2	141.9	150.6
38	85.9	85.7	96.0	111.1	113.9	131.9	137.9
39	75.1	76.4	90.4	100.9	105.4	118.6	127.1
40	67.8	69.9	78.1	90.2	95.0	106.7	115.2
41	62.0	59.7	67.7	74.9	79.6	92.4	100.7
42	50.3	51.1	56.0	63.6	66.9	75.3	83.7
43	40.1	40.1	43.4	52.2	54.3	60.7	63.6
44	29.5	31.5	34.0	39.7	40.8	47.0	48.0
45	21.0	25.2	26.5	29.2	29.7	33.7	37.3
46	16.7	18.1	19.4	20.8	22.5	24.6	24.5
47	13.2	12.9	14.3	15.6	18.4	17.2	17.4
48	9.8	10.6	11.6	13.3	13.3	12.3	14.9
49	8.2	9.3	10.1	10.3	10.2	10.9	11.0
50	8.4	8.5	8.3	8.3	9.7	10.1	8.9
51	8.2	7.8	7.8	8.3	8.5	8.8	9.2
52	6.9	6.9	8.2	7.0	6.7	8.5	8.4
53	6.2	6.5	6.8	6.4	6.0	7.8	6.5
54	2.7	3.2	3.1	3.3	3.1	3.9	2.6
55	0.0	0.0	0.0	0.0	0.0	0.0	0.0
56	0.0	0.0	0.0	0.0	0.0	0.0	0.0
57	0.0	0.0	0.0	0.0	0.0	0.0	0.0
58	0.0	0.0	0.0	0.0	0.0	0.0	0.0
59	0.0	0.0	0.0	0.0	0.0	0.0	0.0
60	0.0	0.0	0.0	0.0	0.0	0.0	0.0
61	0.0	0.0	0.0	0.0	0.0	0.0	0.0
62	0.0	0.0	0.0	0.0	0.0	0.0	0.0
63	0.0	0.0	0.0	0.0	0.0	0.0	0.0
TFR	3,641.5	3,559.2	3,822.5	4,289.0	4,359.6	4,859.5	5,094.3

preceding the census and actual year

7 1972	8 1971	9 1970	10 1969	11 1968	12 1967	13 1966	14 1965
20.4	24.2	26.1	27.4	28.9	28.1	29.6	32.3
46.3	49.9	48.0	50.8	49.5	54.7	57.4	55.4
83.1	81.8	82.0	84.9	87.6	95.8	93.8	89.6
121.7	123.4	122.3	129.8	135.7	141.4	141.6	136.5
161.9	164.2	168.9	176.5	184.9	192.2	191.9	187.5
197.2	205.0	210.2	217.9	233.7	237.7	234.9	233.2
230.8	237.6	244.6	256.8	269.8	277.2	265.6	266.8
248.1	260.6	272.8	282.7	296.3	303.6	286.7	292.5
261.5	282.7	292.0	302.0	310.5	319.1	311.0	314.1
275.3	292.3	305.9	310.7	322.2	328.6	321.4	330.7
273.0	295.4	307.9	309.5	326.6	331.0	321.6	328.7
268.7	290.9	304.5	306.9	322.4	337.1	319.8	329.5
263.9	283.0	298.6	301.4	320.7	328.5	313.4	330.5
256.8	277.0	291.7	294.8	307.0	316.6	308.6	321.5
247.2	269.5	286.8	286.8	295.0	311.7	299.9	317.5
237.6	259.0	268.7	277.3	293.7	303.0	290.4	305.8
227.9	246.0	253.6	266.4	281.3	294.6	278.9	296.5
213.5	236.0	249.5	251.9	270.7	282.4	270.1	290.4
200.2	227.2	235.9	243.6	258.7	274.5	262.0	275.6
194.5	213.9	228.9	235.2	249.3	264.9	250.8	264.6
188.0	208.1	218.0	226.5	242.6	253.0	241.9	252.9
179.0	195.2	206.9	214.7	230.4	238.4	228.3	241.4
165.1	182.9	195.0	198.3	213.8	216.6	214.2	228.9
157.4	173.4	181.1	185.7	194.9	206.8	200.8	207.9
144.3	157.0	163.4	167.2	178.2	195.1	175.8	190.7
124.4	140.0	139.8	145.4	161.6	161.2	153.3	165.0
107.5	120.7	121.4	127.3	134.4	132.3	126.9	134.8
91.0	101.0	104.4	102.0	112.2	108.1	102.8	108.8
71.9	82.6	74.3	77.6	87.0	82.6	82.8	86.0
56.5	57.2	52.1	57.3	59.2	60.9	60.4	65.2
38.2	37.1	38.8	41.9	42.4	44.8	42.9	44.2
25.4	26.4	28.3	28.7	32.0	30.1	28.9	28.4
19.8	20.8	20.0	20.5	22.9	20.3	21.3	23.6
15.5	16.0	16.3	15.1	16.5	15.6	18.2	17.5
13.2	13.6	14.1	13.6	14.3	13.2	14.2	12.1
13.3	11.4	10.5	12.7	13.3	11.5	12.7	0.0
10.5	9.3	9.5	10.7	10.5	9.6	0.0	0.0
7.4	8.6	9.7	9.1	9.2	0.0	0.0	0.0
7.4	8.1	9.2	7.3	0.0	0.0	0.0	0.0
4.4	3.6	5.2	0.0	0.0	0.0	0.0	0.0
0.0	0.0	0.0	0.0	0.0	0.0	0.0	0.0
0.0	0.0	0.0	0.0	0.0	0.0	0.0	0.0
0.0	0.0	0.0	0.0	0.0	0.0	0.0	0.0
0.0	0.0	0.0	0.0	0.0	0.0	0.0	0.0
0.0	0.0	0.0	0.0	0.0	0.0	0.0	0.0
0.0	0.0	0.0	0.0	0.0	0.0	0.0	0.0
0.0	0.0	0.0	0.0	0.0	0.0	0.0	0.0
0.0	0.0	0.0	0.0	0.0	0.0	0.0	0.0
0.0	0.0	0.0	0.0	0.0	0.0	0.0	0.0
5,469.9	5,892.6	6,116.9	6,274.8	6,619.9	6,822.6	6,574.7	6,806.4

126

Table 7.10. Central births, by women's age in five-year age groups, estimated by

							Number of years
Women's age	<1 1979	1 1978	2 1977	3 1976	4 1975	5 1974	6 1973
15–19	1,757	1,629	1,617	1,770	1,666	1,753	1,678
20–24	4,244	3,874	3,879	4,012	3,772	3,933	3,811
25–29	3,241	2,963	2,958	3,110	2,946	3,034	2,992
30–34	1,724	1,587	1,648	1,818	1,859	2,102	2,265
35–39	1,000	1,008	1,127	1,272	1,271	1,382	1,417
40–44	484	471	508	566	577	633	653
45–49	111	118	121	125	127	125	122

Table 7.11. Central woman-years of exposure, by women's age in five-year age Thailand

							Number of years
Women's age	<1 1979	1 1978	2 1977	3 1976	4 1975	5 1974	6 1973
15–19	27,578	26,879	26,362	25,882	25,189	24,162	22,877
20–24	23,878	22,600	21,170	19,665	18,492	17,684	16,841
25–29	17,432	16,593	15,650	14,744	13,771	12,802	12,046
30–34	12,594	11,844	11,325	10,989	10,972	11,065	11,068
35–39	10,859	10,855	10,765	10,589	10,224	9,755	9,459
40–44	9,536	9,240	8,997	8,706	8,411	8,118	7,801
45–49	7,899	7,584	7,201	6,817	6,461	6,009	5,574

applying the own-children method to the 1980 Census: Thailand

preceding the census and actual year

7 1972	8 1971	9 1970	10 1969	11 1968	12 1967	13 1966	14 1965
1,736	1,677	1,605	1,629	1,597	1,568	1,472	1,331
3,820	3,781	3,651	3,524	3,482	3,417	3,225	3,271
3,024	3,171	3,330	3,379	3,548	3,646	3,456	3,477
2,363	2,566	2,594	2,550	2,625	2,683	2,478	2,543
1,543	1,643	1,675	1,666	1,710	1,702	1,547	1,554
681	722	678	656	659	607	551	553
122	116	113	111	113	105	102	98

groups, estimated by applying the own-children method to the 1980 Census:

preceding the census and actual year   ·

7 1972	8 1971	9 1970	10 1969	11 1968	12 1967	13 1966	14 1965
21,438	19,923	18,742	17,932	17,084	16,127	15,206	14,215
15,891	14,978	13,996	13,018	12,255	11,731	11,395	11,390
11,525	11,190	11,178	11,280	11,289	11,208	11,037	10,670
10,982	10,809	10,444	9,971	9,674	9,433	9,140	8,842
9,216	8,924	8,627	8,333	8,013	7,619	7,222	6,855
7,412	7,021	6,659	6,197	5,754	5,403	5,094	4,838
5,231	4,927	4,677	4,500	4,292	4,087	3,964	3,811

Table 7.12. Age-specific central birth rates in five-year age groups, total fertility method to the 1980 Census: Thailand

Rate and Women's age				Number of years			
	<1 1979	1 1978	2 1977	3 1976	4 1975	5 1974	6 1973
ASBR							
15–19	63.7	60.6	61.3	68.4	66.1	72.6	73.4
20–24	177.7	171.4	183.2	204.0	204.0	222.4	226.3
25–29	185.9	178.6	189.0	211.0	214.0	237.0	248.3
30–34	136.9	134.0	145.5	165.4	169.4	189.9	204.6
35–39	92.1	92.9	104.7	120.1	124.3	141.6	149.8
40–44	50.7	51.0	56.5	65.0	68.6	77.9	83.8
45–49	14.1	15.6	16.8	18.4	19.6	20.8	22.0
TFR							
15–49	3,606.1	3,520.4	3,785.5	4,261.4	4,330.0	4,811.3	5,040.9
15–44	3,535.6	3,442.4	3,701.7	4,169.6	4,232.1	4,707.5	4,931.1
GFR							
15–49	114.4	110.3	116.9	130.1	130.6	144.7	151.0
15–44	122.2	117.7	124.5	138.5	138.9	153.6	160.0
STD							
15–49	104.9	102.3	109.9	123.7	125.6	139.6	146.1
15–44	118.7	115.5	124.1	139.7	141.7	157.6	165.0

Note: STD denotes age-standardized GFR.

rates, and general fertility rates, estimated by applying the own-children

preceding the census and actual year

7 1972	8 1971	9 1970	10 1969	11 1968	12 1967	13 1966	14 1965
81.0	84.2	85.7	90.8	93.5	97.2	96.8	93.7
240.4	252.4	260.9	270.7	284.1	291.3	283.0	287.2
262.4	283.4	297.9	299.6	314.3	325.3	313.2	325.8
215.2	237.4	248.4	255.7	271.4	284.4	271.1	287.6
167.4	184.1	194.2	199.9	213.4	223.3	214.2	226.7
91.9	102.9	101.8	105.8	114.6	112.3	108.2	114.3
23.2	23.5	24.1	24.7	26.3	25.6	25.8	25.8
5,407.4	5,839.9	6,065.0	6,236.1	6,587.5	6,797.5	6,561.1	6,805.9
5,291.2	5,722.2	5,944.5	6,112.8	6,455.9	6,669.5	6,432.0	6,676.8
162.7	175.9	183.6	189.7	200.9	209.2	203.5	211.6
172.2	186.2	194.3	200.9	212.6	221.4	215.4	224.1
156.7	169.2	175.7	180.7	190.8	196.9	190.1	197.1
177.0	191.3	198.7	204.3	215.7	222.9	215.0	223.1

Table 7.13. Age-specific central birth rates and total fertility rates for aggregated time periods, estimated by applying the own-children method to the 1980 Census: Thailand

Women's age	Summary rates						
	1965–69	1970–74	1975–79	1967–69	1970–73	1974–76	1977–79
15–19	94.3	78.9	64.0	93.7	80.7	69.0	61.9
20–24	283.0	239.3	187.0	281.7	244.1	209.8	177.3
25–29	315.5	264.8	194.6	313.1	272.5	220.0	184.4
30–34	273.7	218.7	149.6	270.2	226.0	175.0	138.7
35–39	215.0	166.6	106.6	211.9	173.3	128.4	96.5
40–44	110.9	91.0	58.1	110.7	94.7	70.3	52.7
45–49	25.6	22.6	16.7	25.5	23.2	19.5	15.4
TFR (15–49)	6,589.8	5,409.0	3,882.8	6,533.9	5,572.4	4,460.4	3,635.3

Interpolation of Abridged Life Tables to Single Years of Age

In many applications of the own-children method, especially in developing countries, life tables by single years of age are not available, so that it is necessary to interpolate abridged life tables to single years of age. This appendix describes procedures developed by Feeney (1974) for interpolating abridged life table survival proportions, $\ell_0, \ell_1, \ell_5, \ell_{10}, \ell_{15}, \ldots,$ ℓ_{85}, to survival proportions by single years of age, $\ell_0, \ell_1, \ell_2, \ell_3, \ell_4, \ldots,$ ℓ_{84}, ℓ_{85} (see also Retherford 1978). The procedure is in four parts, pertaining to four age ranges. The first is for ages 1–4, the second for ages 5–9, the third for ages 10 to the lower boundary of the last five-year age group (80 in this case), and the fourth for the last five-year age group (80–84 in this case). The procedure does not depend on the last age in the abridged life table. Therefore, the same interpolation coefficients in Table A.1, presented later, can be used even when the age at which the open age interval begins is an age other than 85 (say, 75). Here we assume that the abridged life table terminates at age 85.

Interpolation of ages 1–4

We are given ℓ_1 and ℓ_5 and would like interpolated values of ℓ_2, ℓ_3, and ℓ_4. Polynomial interpolation is unsatisfactory because it does not adequately capture the unusual curvature of the ℓ_x curve owing to rapidly declining ℓ_x in the second year of life followed by much more slowly declining ℓ_x at subsequent ages. We therefore make recourse to a regression procedure developed by Coale and Demeny (1966:20–23).

According to this method, weights a_2, a_3, and a_4 are determined so that $\ell_x = a_x \ell_1 + (1 - a_x)\ell_5$. Values of a_x are given by Coale and Demeny for each of the four model life table families (West, North, East, and South). When $q_0 \geqslant 0.100$, constant values of a_2, a_3, and a_4 are used, and when $q_0 < 0.100$, variable weights a_x^* are used, of the form $a_x^* = a_x + b_x(0.1 - q_0)$. For the West region, the values of a_2, a_3, and a_4 are 0.489, 0.260, and

0.112 for females and 0.484, 0.258, and 0.110 for males. The values of b_2, b_3, and b_4 are 0.656, 0.601, and 0.370 for females and 1.353, 1.089, and 0.571 for males.

Interpolation of ages 6–9

A matrix approach to polynomial interpolation is used for the age group 6–9 (Feeney 1974; Retherford 1978). The basic idea of the procedure is to fit a cubic polynomial through the abridged ℓ_x values ℓ_4 (as determined by the procedure in the previous section), ℓ_5, ℓ_{10}, and ℓ_{15} and then to read values of ℓ_6, ℓ_7, ℓ_8, and ℓ_9 from the fitted curve. The form of the curve is

$$\ell_x = a_0 + a_1x + a_2x^2 + a_3x^3. \tag{A.1}$$

(Although the same notation is used, the coefficients a_x in this equation are unrelated to the weights a_x of the previous section.)

To simplify the problem we first translate ages by subtracting five from all ages. Age 5 then becomes age 0. This coordinate transformation has no effect on the ultimate result; indeed, any number could be subtracted from each age without affecting the final outcome. We shall retain, however, the original untranslated ages as subscripts of the ℓ's.

It then follows from equation (A.1) that

$$\ell_4 = a_0 + a_1(-1) + a_2(-1)^2 + a_3(-1)^3$$

$$\ell_5 = a_0$$

$$\ell_{10} = a_0 + a_1(5) + a_2(5)^2 + a_3(5)^3 \tag{A.2}$$

$$\ell_{15} = a_0 + a_1(10) + a_2(10)^2 + a_3(10)^3.$$

In matrix notation, equations (A.2) may be written

$$\ell_G = C_0\,A, \tag{A.3}$$

where ℓ_G (subscript G denoting given) is the column vector,

$$\ell_G = \begin{pmatrix} \ell_4 \\ \ell_5 \\ \ell_{10} \\ \ell_{15} \end{pmatrix}, \tag{A.4}$$

C_0 is the matrix of coefficients,

$$C_0 = \begin{pmatrix} 1 & -1 & 1 & -1 \\ 1 & 0 & 0 & 0 \\ 1 & 5 & 25 & 125 \\ 1 & 10 & 100 & 1000 \end{pmatrix}, \tag{A.5}$$

and A is the column vector

$$A = \begin{pmatrix} a_0 \\ a_1 \\ a_2 \\ a_3 \end{pmatrix} . \tag{A.6}$$

If the value of A is known, we may obtain interpolated single-year values of ℓ_x from equation (2.13) as follows:

$$\begin{aligned} \ell_6 &= a_0 + a_1(1) + a_2(1)^2 + a_3(1)^3 \\ \ell_7 &= a_0 + a_1(2) + a_2(2)^2 + a_3(2)^3 \\ \ell_8 &= a_0 + a_1(3) + a_2(3)^2 + a^3(3)^3 \\ \ell_9 &= a_0 + a_1(4) + a_2(4)^2 + a_3(4)^3, \end{aligned} \tag{A.7}$$

which can be written in matrix form as

$$\ell_I = C_1 A \tag{A.8}$$

(subscript I denoting interpolated), where the three quantities in this equation are defined in a way parallel to equations (A.4) through (A.6).

If we denote the matrix inverse of C_0 as C_0^{-1}, we may combine equations (A.3) and (A.8) to give

$$\ell_I = (C_1 C_0^{-1}) \ell_G. \tag{A.9}$$

If we denote the matrix of multipliers $(C_1 C_0^{-1})$ simply as M, then equation (A.9) can be written even more simply as

$$\ell_I = M \ell_G. \tag{A.10}$$

The matrix M of multipliers is easily calculated, since C_0 is of a simple numerical form given by equation (A.5) and C_1 of an equally simple form given as the matrix of numerical coefficients of equations (A.7). The first panel of Table A.1 gives the M matrix for this age group.

Interpolation of ages 11–79

To interpolate ages 11–79 we fit the cubic in equation (A.1) through ℓ_{x-5}, ℓ_x, ℓ_{x+5}, and ℓ_{x+10}, for $x = 5, 10, \ldots, 75$ and thus obtain values of ℓ_{x+1}, ℓ_{x+2}, ℓ_{x+3}, and ℓ_{x+4} from the fitted curve.

To simplify the computations we first translate ages by subtracting x from all ages, so that x becomes age 0. As before, the translation has no effect on the result. We again retain the original untranslated ages as subscripts of the ℓ's.

It then follows from equation (A.1) that

$$\ell_{x-5} = a_0 + a_1(-5) + a_2(-5)^2 + a_3(-5)^3$$
$$\ell_x = a_0$$
$$\ell_{x+5} = a_0 + a_1(5) + a_2(5)^2 + a_3(5)^3 \tag{A.11}$$
$$\ell_{x+10} = a_0 + a_1(10) + a_2(10)^2 + a_3(10)^3,$$

which can again be written in matrix notation as

$$\ell_G = \mathbf{C_0\,A}. \tag{A.12}$$

We have also

$$\ell_{x+1} = a_0 + a_1(1) + a_2(1)^2 + a_3(1)^3$$
$$\ell_{x+2} = a_0 + a_1(2) + a_2(2)^2 + a_3(2)^3$$
$$\ell_{x+3} = a_0 + a_1(3) + a_2(3)^2 + a_3(3)^3 \tag{A.13}$$
$$\ell_{x+4} = a_0 + a_1(4) + a_2(4)^2 + a_3(4)^3,$$

which can again be written in matrix notation as

$$\ell_I = \mathbf{C_1\,A}. \tag{A.14}$$

Equations (A.12) and (A.14) can be combined as before to give equation (A.10).

Although the same notation is used in equations (A.12) and (A.14) as in equations (A.3) and (A.8), the quantities symbolized in the two cases are of course different and should not be confused. Identical notation is used both to highlight similarities in underlying logic and to achieve economy in presentation. The midpanel of Table A.1 gives the $\mathbf{M}$ matrix for this age group.

Table A.1. Multiplier matrices for interpolation of abridged life tables to complete life tables

First panel	−0.545455	1.440000	0.120000	−0.014545
	−0.727273	1.440000	0.320000	−0.032727
	−0.636364	1.120000	0.560000	−0.043636
	−0.363636	0.600000	0.800000	−0.036364
Midpanel	−0.048000	0.864000	0.216000	−0.032000
	−0.064000	0.672000	0.448000	−0.056000
	−0.056000	0.448000	0.672000	−0.064000
	−0.032000	0.216000	0.864000	−0.048000
End panel	0.032000	−0.176000	1.056000	0.088000
	0.056000	−0.288000	1.008000	0.224000
	0.064000	−0.312000	0.832000	0.416000
	0.048000	−0.224000	0.504000	0.672000

Note: The first panel of multipliers is used to compute interpolated values of ℓ_x for ages 6–9, the end panel for the last age group, and the midpanel for the ages in the middle. The multiplier matrices are unaffected by the age at which the abridged life table terminates. Each panel of multipliers corresponds to the matrix $\mathbf{M}$ in equation (A.10).

Interpolation of ages 81–84

For the interpolation of ages 81–84 we fit the cubic in equation (1) through ℓ_{70}, ℓ_{75}, ℓ_{80}, and ℓ_{85} and obtain interpolated values of ℓ_{81}, ℓ_{82}, ℓ_{83}, and ℓ_{84} from the fitted curve. Age 80 is translated to age 0. We have

$$\ell_{70} = a_0 + a_1(-10) + a_2(-10)^2 + a_3(-10)^3$$
$$\ell_{75} = a_0 + a_1(-5) + a_2(-5)^2 + a_3(-5)^3$$
$$\ell_{80} = a_0 \qquad\qquad\qquad\qquad\qquad\qquad\qquad (A.15)$$
$$\ell_{85} = a_0 + a_1(5) + a_2(5)^2 + a_3(5)^3$$

and

$$\ell_{81} = a_0 + a_1(1) + a_2(1)^2 + a_3(1)^3$$
$$\ell_{82} = a_0 + a_1(2) + a_2(2)^2 + a_3(2)^3$$
$$\ell_{83} = a_0 + a_1(3) + a_2(3)^2 + a_3(3)^3 \qquad\qquad (A.16)$$
$$\ell_{84} = a_0 + a_1(4) + a_2(4)^2 + a_3(4)^3.$$

Again these two sets of equations may be reduced to the form of equation (A.10) by the logic described in the previous two sections. Note that the end panel of multipliers in Table A.1 obtained by this procedure is the same even if the life table ends at an age other than 85. This is true because the matrices C_0 and C_1 are unaffected by the age at which the abridged life table is terminated.

Sampling Variability of
Own-Children Fertility Estimates

Under certain simplifying assumptions it is possible to derive approximation formulas for the standard errors of own-children estimates of age-
specific birth rates and total fertility rates (Retherford and Bennett
1977). We consider only the case in which age-specific birth rates for
women in five-year age groups are estimated for single calendar years.
Some additional notation is needed:

$_5U_a^w$: Adjustment factor for underenumeration of women aged a to $a + 5$

$_5F_a(t)$: Central age-specific birth rate for women aged a to $a + 5$ in year t to $t + 1$

TFR(t) : Total fertility rate in year t to $t + 1$, computed as $5 \sum {_5}F_a(t)$, where the summation ranges over five-year age groups

$_5C_{x,a}$: Number of enumerated own children aged x to $x + 1$ of mothers aged a to $a + 5$

$_5\tilde{C}_{x,a}$: Number of enumerated own children aged x to $x + 1$ of mothers aged a to $a + 5$, adjusted for underenumeration and age misreporting and for non-own children as $_5C_{x,a} U_x^c V_x$ (in this latter expression, U_x^c is used in place of $U_{x,a}^c$ to simplify the derivations that follow)

$_5W_a$: Number of enumerated women aged a to $a + 5$

$_5\tilde{W}_a$: Number of enumerated women aged a to $a + 5$, adjusted for underenumeration and age misreporting as $_5W_a {_5}U_a^w$

$_5H_{x,a}$: Age-specific child–woman ratio, $_5\tilde{C}_{x,a}/{_5}\tilde{W}_a$

$_5R_{a \leftarrow b}$: Reverse-survival factor, from age group b to $b + 5$ to age group a to $a + 5$. Defined as in Chapter 2, except that the L's are for five-year age groups instead of single-year age groups (formulas are unchanged, except that a subscript 5 is inserted in front of each L).

Other notation is as previously defined. With enumeration at time t, age-specific birth rates for five-year age groups of women can then be calculated as

$$_5F_a(t - x - 1) = \{.5[_5\tilde{C}_{\cdot,a+x} + _5\tilde{C}_{\cdot,a+x+1}]r_{0\leftarrow x}\}/$$
$$\{.5[_5\tilde{W}_{a+x} + _5\tilde{W}_{a+x+1}]R^f_{a\leftarrow a+x+.5}\}. \tag{B.1}$$

As explained earlier, rates are actually calculated by reverse-surviving both women and children by single years of age and then aggregating reverse-survived women into five-year age groups. But for purposes of deriving formulas for standard errors, it is convenient to begin with the slightly cruder approximation given by equation (B.1).

We have that

$$\{.5[_5\tilde{C}_{x,a+x} + _5\tilde{C}_{x,a+x+1}]\}/\{.5[_5\tilde{W}_{a+x} + _5\tilde{W}_{a+x+1}]\}$$
$$\cong {_5\tilde{C}_{x,a+x+.5}}/{_5\tilde{W}_{a+x+.5}} = {_5H_{x,a+x+.5}}. \tag{B.2}$$

Hence, equation (2.14) can be rewritten as

$$_5F_a(t - x - 1) = {_5H_{x,a+x+.5}}[r_{0\leftarrow x}/{_5R^f_{a\leftarrow a+x+.5}}] \tag{B.3}$$

or, even more simply, as

$$F = k H, \tag{B.4}$$

where k denotes the quotient of reverse-survival ratios on the right-hand side of equation (B.3), and time and age values are understood.

For purposes of calculating standard errors, we treat k as constant and $H = \tilde{C}/\tilde{W}$ as a random variable. The justification for treating the mortality function k as constant is that the variance of k is generally quite small, since k is very close to one in most own-children applications. (The reverse-survival ratios themselves are each close to one, and the ratio of one to the other is even closer to one.) The age-specific child–woman ratio, H, can be viewed as the proportion of sample women in a five-year age group who have a child aged x to $x + 1$. Thus the problems of determining the standard error of the age-specific birth rate, F, in equation (B.4) can be reduced to the simpler problem of determining the sampling error of the proportion H.

We assume that the sample of households from the census or household survey approximates a simple random sample of women. If clustering is minimal, this assumption seems justified. The sampling distribution of F in equation (B.4) is then approximated by the usual distribution of F in simple random samples, with standard error equal to k times the standard error of H,

$$s_F = k\{[(1 - f)H(1 - H)]/(\tilde{W} - 1)\}^{.5}, \tag{B.5}$$

where f is the sampling fraction and $\tilde{W}$ is the denominator of the proportion $H = \tilde{C}/\tilde{W}$. This formula derives from the usual formula for the standard error of a sample proportion, P, namely $s_p = [P(1 - P)/N]^{.5}$. The term $(1 - f)$ is a finite population correction (Cochran 1963:60) that should be included when the sample is a census sample because the sampling fraction is then typically 5 percent or more. Note that F can be substituted for H in (B.5) without much loss of accuracy, thereby simplifying the calculations. Equation (B.5) then simplifies to

$$s_F = k\{[(1 - f)F(1 - F)]/(\tilde{W} - 1)\}^{.5}. \tag{B.6}$$

Given estimated standard errors and confidence intervals of age-specific birth rates for a given year, we can calculate the estimated standard error and confidence interval of the total fertility rate for that year as

$$s_{TFR} = 5(\Sigma_i s_{F_i}^2)^{.5}, \tag{B.7}$$

where F_i is the ith age-specific birth rate. An underlying assumption of equation (B.7) is that the covariance between any two age-specific birth rates is zero. Since the age-specific birth rates on which the TFR is based are cross-sectional, with each rate based on a largely different birth cohort of women, the assumption of zero covariance seems justified. There is some overlap of birth cohorts at the end of each age interval and the beginning of the next, but we assume that it can be safely ignored. Work by William Brass (1976) on a simple birth distribution model incorporating the relevant dependencies suggests that the assumption of independence gives standard errors and confidence intervals close enough to the true ones for practical purposes.

If age-specific birth rates are approximately known in advance (e.g., from estimates from an earlier period or from a similar population where fertility is known), it is a simple matter to obtain a rough estimate of the minimum sample size (persons, not households) needed in order that the 95 percent confidence interval about an age-specific birth rate be no more than, say, ±10 percent of that rate. We simply express s_F, as given in equation (B.5), as a function of overall sample size S and then solve the equation

$$(1.96 s_F)/F = .1 \tag{B.8}$$

for S (1.96 being the 95 percent cutoff point under the assumption that the sampling distribution is normal). Since the calculation of the standard error is rather rough to begin with, the calculation of S can be further simplified by setting $k = 1$, substituting F for H, and using $\tilde{W}$ in place of $\tilde{W} - 1$ in (B.5). Let d denote the ratio of the adjusted number of sample women in the age group to total sample size, $\tilde{W}/S$, so that $\tilde{W} = d\,S$. (Typical values of d can be obtained from, say, the previous census.) Then (B.8) becomes

$$\{1.96[F(1 - F)/(d\,S)]^{.5}\}/F = .1, \tag{B.9}$$

implying that

$$S = 384\,(1 - F)/(F\,d). \tag{B.10}$$

Similarly, if our criterion is that

$$(1.96\,s_{TFR})/\text{TFR} = .1, \tag{B.11}$$

it is easily demonstrated that

$$S = 9604(1/\text{TFR}^2)\Sigma_i\,[F_i(1 - F_i)/d_i], \tag{B.12}$$

where the summation is over five-year age groups in the reproductive age range. In (B.10) and (B.12) both F_i and TFR are expressed on a per-woman basis, not on a per-thousand basis. In the case of own-children estimates of fertility derived from the 1970 Census of the Philippines, it was found that a sample size of about 10,000 was necessary to meet the criterion specified by equation (B.11) for the TFR (Retherford and Bennett 1977: table 3).

Equations (B.5) to (B.12) assume that the size of a given sample subgroup (as defined by age or other characteristics) is a fixed constant over repeated samples, not a random variable. Treatment of sample subgroup size as a random variable would slightly increase the estimated sampling variability. Treatment of reverse-survival ratios as random variables would have a similar effect, as would also abandonment of the assumption of simple random sampling. For all these reasons, equations (B.5) to (B.12) provide minimum estimates of standard errors, confidence intervals, and required sample sizes. If the sample is of enumeration districts rather than households, design effects from clustering can no longer be ignored, and standard errors, confidence intervals, and required sample sizes may be substantially larger than values computed by the formulas given here.

Selected Computer Programs

The computer programs for the own-children method in use at the East–West Population Institute have been developed in three modules corresponding to the three stages described in Chapter 7. Each module can be used either independently or successively. In this appendix, the computer programs for the three stages are described and listings of selected programs are reproduced. The programs are designed to run on a large computer with magnetic tape units. Two new versions of the computer programs are under development. The first is a simplified but more completely packaged set of programs. (Some of the current programs require modification for each new data set.) The second is an even more streamlined version suitable for microcomputers. The current version of the complete three-stage computer program package for the own-children method with documentation may be obtained by writing to

Supervisory Computer Specialist
East–West Population Institute
East–West Center
1777 East–West Road
Honolulu, Hawaii 96848, U.S.A.

MATCH

The program called MATCH matches women with their own children. The input is a set of records on a person-by-person basis grouped by households. The output is a set of records of two types. The first type is a separate record for each woman between the ages of 15 and 65. This record contains the characteristics of the woman and the age and sex of each of her own children who are present in the household. The second type is a record for each household containing unmatched (i.e., non-own) children under age 15. This record contains the age, sex, and relationship to household head of each non-own child in the household.

The program is written in PL/I computer language. In the version of the program presented in Listing C.1, the census to which the program was applied (the Republic of Korea's 1980 Census) collected detailed information on number of living children. For each woman the number of male and of female children living in the same household (MLH and FLH) was collected, and these numbers were used as maximum possible numbers of own children of each sex who could be matched to that woman. When such detailed information is not available, the total number of living children or the total number of children ever born may be used instead without affecting the accuracy of the matching by very much. The input and output record layouts used by the program are shown in Figure C.1.

Listing C.1. MATCH

```
00000010 STAGE1: PROC OPTIONS(MAIN);
00000020 DCL INFILE RECORD SEQUENTIAL BUFFERED INPUT
00000030   ENV(CONSECUTIVE FB RECSIZE(37) BLKSIZE(3700) TOTAL),
00000040      OUTF   RECORD SEQUENTIAL BUFFERED OUTPUT
00000050   ENV(CONSECUTIVE FB RECSIZE(83) BLKSIZE(8300) TOTAL);
00000060 DCL 1 INDATA,
00000070   2 TYPE   CHAR(1),      /* CC.  1     */
00000080   2 ID     CHAR(16),     /*      2-17 */
00000090   2 LINENO CHAR(3),      /*     18-20 */
00000100   2 REL    CHAR(1),      /*     21     */
00000110   2 FILL0  CHAR(1),      /*     22     */
00000120   2 SEX    CHAR(1),      /*     23     */
00000130   2 FILL1  CHAR(1),      /*     24     */
00000140   2 AGE    PIC'99',      /*     25-26 */
00000150   2 MS     CHAR(1),      /*     27     */
00000160   2 AGEFM  PIC'99',      /*     28-29 */
00000170   2 MLH    PIC'9',       /*     30     */
00000180   2 FLH    PIC'9',       /*     31     */
00000190   2 FILL2  CHAR(6);      /*     32-37 */
00000200
00000210 DCL 1 WOMEN(150),
00000220   2 TYPE   CHAR(1),      /* CC.  1     */
00000230   2 ID     CHAR(16),     /*      2-17 */
00000240   2 LINENO CHAR(3),      /*     18-20 */
00000250   2 REL    CHAR(1),      /*     21     */
00000260   2 FILL0  CHAR(1),      /*     22     */
00000270   2 SEX    CHAR(1),      /*     23     */
00000280   2 FILL1  CHAR(1),      /*     24     */
00000290   2 AGE    PIC'99',      /*     25-26 */
00000300   2 MS     CHAR(1),      /*     27     */
00000310   2 AGEFM  PIC'99',      /*     28-29 */
00000320   2 MLH    PIC'9',       /*     30     */
00000330   2 FLH    PIC'9',       /*     31     */
00000340   2 FILL2  CHAR(6);      /*     32-37 */
00000350
00000360 DCL 1 SONS(30),
00000370   2 REL CHAR(1),    2 AGE PIC'99',   2 SEX CHAR(1),
00000380
00000390      1 DAUGH(30),
00000400   2 REL CHAR(1),    2 AGE PIC'99',   2 SEX CHAR(1);
00000410
00000420 DCL 1 OUTO,
```

Listing C.1. MATCH *(continued)*

```
00000430  2 OTYPE CHAR(1),           /* CC.   1     */
00000440  2 WOMDAT,
00000450  3 TYPE   CHAR(1),          /*        2    */
00000460  3 ID      CHAR(16),        /*       3-18  */
00000470  3 LINENO CHAR(3),          /*      19-21  */
00000480  3 REL    CHAR(1),          /*      22     */
00000490  3 FILL0  CHAR(1),          /*      23     */
00000500  3 SEX    CHAR(1),          /*      24     */
00000510  3 FILL1  CHAR(1),          /*      25     */
00000520  3 AGE    PIC'99',          /*      26-27  */
00000530  3 MS     CHAR(1),          /*      28     */
00000540  3 AGEFM  PIC'99',          /*      29-30  */
00000550  3 MLH    PIC'9',           /*      31     */
00000560  3 FLH    PIC'9',           /*      32     */
00000570  3 FILL2  CHAR(6),          /*      33-38  */
00000580  2 KIDDAT(15),              /*      39-83  */
00000590  3 AGE PIC'99',      3 SEX CHAR(1);
00000600
00000610 DCL 1 NONOWN,
00000620    2 NTYPE CHAR(1),
00000630    2 TYPE  CHAR(1),
00000640    2 ID    CHAR(16),
00000650    2 BLANKS CHAR(20),
00000660    2 KIDS(15),
00000670    3 AGE PIC'99',     3 SEX CHAR(1);
00000680
00000690 DCL 1 O_NULL,
00000700    2 OTYPE CHAR(1) INIT(' '),
00000710    2 WOMDAT,
00000720    3 TYPE   CHAR(1) INIT(' '),
00000730    3 ID     CHAR(16) INIT((16) ' '),
00000740    3 LINENO CHAR(3) INIT((3) ' '),
00000750    3 REL    CHAR(1) INIT(' '),
00000760    3 FILL0  CHAR(1) INIT(' '),
00000770    3 SEX    CHAR(1) INIT(' '),
00000780    3 FILL1  CHAR(1) INIT(' '),
00000790    3 AGE    PIC'99' INIT(0),
00000800    3 MS     CHAR(1) INIT(' '),
00000810    3 AGEFM  PIC'99' INIT(0),
00000820    3 MLH    PIC'9' INIT('0'),
00000830    3 FLH    PIC'9' INIT('0'),
00000840    2 KIDDAT(15),
00000850    3 AGE PIC'99' INIT((15) 99),  3 SEX CHAR(1) INIT((15)(1) '9');
00000860
00000870 DCL 1 N_NULL,
00000880    2 NTYPE CHAR(1) INIT(' '),
00000890    2 TYPE  CHAR(1) INIT(' '),
00000900    2 ID    CHAR(16) INIT((16) ' '),
00000910    2 BLANKS CHAR(20) INIT((20) ' '),
00000920    2 KIDS(15),
00000930    3 AGE PIC'99' INIT((15) 99),   3 SEX CHAR(1) INIT((15)(1)'9');
00000940
00000950 /*
00000960   DECLARE RELATIONSHIP TO HEAD VARIABLES AND INITIALIZE THEM
00000970   TO THE CORRESPONDING RELATIONSHIP CODE.
00000980 */
00000990  DCL HEAD CHAR(1) INIT('1'),
00001000      SPOUSE CHAR(1) INIT('2'),
00001010      CHILD_OF_HEAD CHAR(1) INIT('3'),
00001020      OTHER_RELATIVE CHAR(1) INIT('4'),
00001030      NON_RELATIVE  CHAR(1) INIT('5');
00001040
00001050 /*
00001060 NOW DECLARE COUNTERS TO BE USED, FIRST PER HOUSEH, THEN FOR RUN  */
00001070    DCL (NSON, NDAUG, NWOM, REMSON, REMDAU, NKIDO, NONO)
00001080        FIXED BIN;
```

Listing C.1. MATCH *(continued)*

```
00001090        DCL (IREC, NHOUS, WREC, NONREC, MATCD, TNONK)
00001100            FIXED(31,0) BIN;
00001110        DCL SAVEH CHAR(16);
00001120        ON ENDFILE (INFILE) GO TO PAU;
00001130 /*
00001140 GET THINGS STARTED   */
00001150        NHOUS,WREC,NONREC,MATCD,TNONK = 0;
00001160        CALL BLANK;
00001170        READ FILE(INFILE) INTO(INDATA);
00001180        SAVEH = INDATA.ID;      IREC = 1;
00001190        CALL PLACE;
00001200 /*
00001210 MAIN LOOP      */
00001220 NEXT:
00001230        READ FILE(INFILE) INTO(INDATA);
00001240        IREC = IREC + 1;
00001250        IF SAVEH = INDATA.ID THEN CALL PLACE;
00001260        ELSE DO;
00001270                NHOUS = NHOUS + 1;
00001280                CALL MATCH;
00001290                SAVEH = INDATA.ID;
00001300                CALL BLANK;
00001310                CALL PLACE;
00001320                END;
00001330        GO TO NEXT;
00001340 /*
00001350 END IT ALL   */
00001360 PAU:
00001370        NHOUS = NHOUS + 1;
00001380        CALL MATCH;
00001390        CALL TALOUT;
000014001PLACE:
00001410            PROCEDURE;
00001420 /*
00001430 THIS ROUTINE PLACES DATA AS FOLLOWS AND KEEPS A TALLY
00001440        (1) POTENTIAL SONS IN SONS
00001450        (2) WOMEN AGES 15-65 IN WOMEN
00001460        (3) POTENTIAL DAUGHTER IN DAUGH    */
00001470
00001480        IF INDATA.SEX = '1' THEN DO;
00001490                        IF INDATA.AGE>='00' & INDATA.AGE<'15' THEN
00001500                                    CALL SSON;
00001510                        END;
00001520        ELSE DO;
00001530                IF INDATA.AGE>='00' & INDATA.AGE < '15' THEN CALL SDAU
00001540                IF INDATA.AGE >'14' & INDATA.AGE < '66' THEN CALL SFEM
00001550            END;
00001560
00001570 SSON:
00001580        PROCEDURE;
00001590        NSON = NSON + 1;
00001600        SONS(NSON) = INDATA, BY NAME;
00001610        IF INDATA.AGE < '15' THEN REMSON = REMSON + 1;
00001620        END SSON;
00001630
00001640 SDAU:
00001650        PROCEDURE;
00001660        NDAUG = NDAUG + 1;
00001670        DAUGH(NDAUG) = INDATA, BY NAME;
00001680        IF INDATA.AGE < '15' THEN REMDAU = REMDAU + 1;
00001690        END SDAU;
00001700
00001710 SFEM:
00001720        PROCEDURE;
00001730        DCL (C_A, A_F_M) FIXED BIN;
00001740        NWOM = NWOM + 1;
```

Listing C.1. MATCH *(continued)*

```
00001750        WOMEN(NWOM) = INDATA, BY NAME;
00001760        END SFEM;
00001770        END PLACE;
000017801MATCH:
00001790          PROCEDURE;
00001800          DCL IW FIXED BIN;
00001810  /*
00001820     AN OUTPUT RECORD IS WRITTEN FOR EACH WOMAN.
00001830     IF SHE HAS KIDS AN ATTEMPT TO FIND HER KIDS IS MADE.
00001840     WHEN ALL WOMEN HAVE BEEN PROCESSED, NON-OWN KIDS, IF ANY, WILL
00001850     BE WRITTEN      */
00001860
00001870     IF NWOM > 0 THEN
00001880                DO IW = 1 TO NWOM;
00001890                OUTO = O_NULL, BY NAME;
00001900                OUTO.OTYPE = '1';
00001910                NKIDO = 0;
00001920                OUTO.WOMDAT = WOMEN(IW), BY NAME;
00001930
00001940     IF WOMEN.MLH(IW)>'0' & WOMEN.MLH(IW)<='9'
00001950                THEN CALL FKID(SONS,NSON,REMSON,'1');
00001960     IF WOMEN.FLH(IW)>'0' & WOMEN.FLH(IW)<='9'
00001970                THEN CALL FKID(DAUGH,NDAUG,REMDAU,'2');
00001980     WRITE FILE(OUTF) FROM(OUTO);
00001990     WREC = WREC + 1;
00002000     END;
00002010
00002020     /*
00002030     NOW SEE IF ANY-UNMATCHED KIDS */
00002040     IF (REMSON + REMDAU) >0 THEN
00002050        DO;
00002060        NONOWN = N_NULL, BY NAME; NONOWN.NTYPE='2';
00002070        NONOWN.TYPE='1';    NONOWN.ID=SAVEH;
00002080        IF REMSON > 0 THEN CALL ORPH(SONS,NSON,'1',REMSON);
00002090        IF REMDAU > 0 THEN CALL ORPH(DAUGH,NDAUG,'2',REMDAU);
00002100        WRITE FILE(OUTF) FROM(NONOWN);
00002110        NONREC = NONREC + 1;
00002120        END;
000021301FKID:
00002140          PROCEDURE (CHILD,NCHILD,NLEFT,ISEX);
00002150          DCL 1 CHILD(30) CONNECTED,
00002160             2 CREL CHAR(1),      2 CAGE PIC '99',   2 CSEX CHAR(1),
00002170           (NCHILD,NLEFT,IWAGE) FIXED BIN,
00002180           ISEX CHAR(1),   (CHD,KHOME)   FIXED BIN,
00002190           TREL CHAR(1);
00002200  /*
00002210  THIS ROUTINE SEARCHES FOR KIDS.  IF THE KID IS LESS THAN 15,
00002220  IT GETS PUT INTO THE OUTPUT AREA. WHEN KIDS ARE FOUND THEIR
00002230  RELATIONSHIPS ARE DUMMIED TO PREVENT FURTHUR MATCH   */
00002240
00002250     IF NLEFT > 0 THEN
00002260        DO;
00002270        TREL = WOMEN.REL(IW);       IWAGE = WOMEN.AGE(IW);
00002280        IF ISEX='1' THEN KHOME = WOMEN.MLH(IW);
00002290                    ELSE KHOME = WOMEN.FLH(IW);
00002300  /*
00002310  LOOP PER KID */
00002320     DO CHD = 1 TO NCHILD WHILE (KHOME > 0);
00002330     IF (TREL=HEAD | TREL=SPOUSE) & CREL(CHD)=CHILD_OF_HEAD THEN
00002340        CALL CHECK;               /* MATCH FEMALE HEAD OR SPOUSE OF HEAD TO
00002350                                        CHILD OF HEAD      */
00002360     ELSE IF TREL=CHILD_OF_HEAD & CREL(CHD)=OTHER_RELATIVE THEN
00002370        CALL CHECK;            /* MATCH DAUGHTER OF HEAD TO HER CHILDREN   */
00002380     ELSE IF TREL=OTHER_RELATIVE & CREL(CHD)=OTHER_RELATIVE THEN
00002390        CALL CHECK;   /* MATCH OTHER FEMALE RELATIVE TO HER CHILDREN */
00002400     ELSE IF TREL=NON_RELATIVE & CREL(CHD)=NON_RELATIVE THEN
```

Listing C.1. MATCH *(continued)*

```
00002410 CALL CHECK;      ‾ /* MATCH FEMALE NON-RELATIVE TO HER CHILDREN    */
00002420        END;
00002430        END;
00002440
0000245O1CHECK:
00002460        PROCEDURE;
00002470 /*
00002480 THIS CHECKS IF THE AGE DIFFERENCE B/W MOM AND KID IS B/W 15 AND 49.
00002490 ALSO, IF KID'S AGE IS < 15, IS PLACED IN OUTA  */
00002500
00002510        DCL KSEX CHAR(1);
00002520            KAGE = CAGE(CHD);    IDF = IWAGE-KAGE;    KSEX=CSEX(CHD);
00002530            IF IDF > 14 & IDF < 50 THEN
00002540                DO;
00002550                IF KAGE < 15 THEN DO;
00002560                            NKIDO = NKIDO + 1;
00002570                            MATCD = MATCD + 1;
00002580                            OUTO.KIDDAT(NKIDO).AGE=KAGE;
00002590                            OUTO.KIDDAT(NKIDO).SEX=KSEX;
00002600                            NLEFT = NLEFT - 1;
00002610                            END;
00002620                KHOME = KHOME - 1;
00002630                CREL(CHD) = 'X';
00002640                END;
00002650        END CHECK;
00002660        END FKID;
0000267O1ORPH:
00002680        PROCEDURE(CHILD,NCHILD,ISEX,REM);
00002690 /*
00002700    THIS MOVES UNMATCHED KIDS TO OUTA AND COUNTS THEM  */
00002710
00002720        DCL  1 CHILD(30) CONNECTED,
00002730            2    REL  CHAR(1),  2  AGE PIC '99',   2 SEX CHAR(1),
00002740            NCHILD FIXED BIN,   ISEX CHAR(1),   REM FIXED BIN;
00002750        DO I = 1 TO NCHILD WHILE (REM > 0);
00002760        IF REL(I)  ‾= 'X' & AGE(I) < 15 THEN
00002770            DO; REM = REM - 1;
00002780                NONO = NONO + 1;  TNONK = TNONK + 1;
00002790                NONOWN.KIDS(NONO) = CHILD(I), BY NAME;
00002800            END;
00002810        END;
00002820
00002830        END ORPH;
00002840        END MATCH;
0000285O1BLANK:
00002860        PROCEDURE;
00002870 /*
00002880 THIS JUST INITIALIZES COUNTERS AND AREAS ON A PER-HOUSEHOLD BASIS */
00002890        NSON,NDAUG,NWOM,REMSON,REMDAU,NKIDO,NONO = 0;
00002900        END BLANK;
00002910  TALOUT:
00002920        PROCEDURE;
00002930 /*
00002940    THIS SIMPLY PRINTS COUNTER INFO   */
00002950        PUT PAGE EDIT ('NO OF RECORDS READ ', IREC) (A,F(10));
00002960        PUT EDIT ('NO OF WOMEN OUTPUT ', WREC,
00002970                  'NO OF NON-OWN RECORDS ', NONREC,
00002980                  'NO OF HOUSEHOLDS ',NHOUS,
00002990                  'NO OF MATCHED KIDS ', MATCD,
00003000                  'NO OF NON-OWN KIDS ', TNONK)
00003010         (5 (COL(1), A, F(6)) );
00003020        WREC = WREC + NONREC;
00003030        PUT EDIT ('TOTAL NO OF OUTPUT RECORDS',WREC) (COL(1),A,F(6));
00003040        END TALOUT;
00003050        END STAGE1;
```

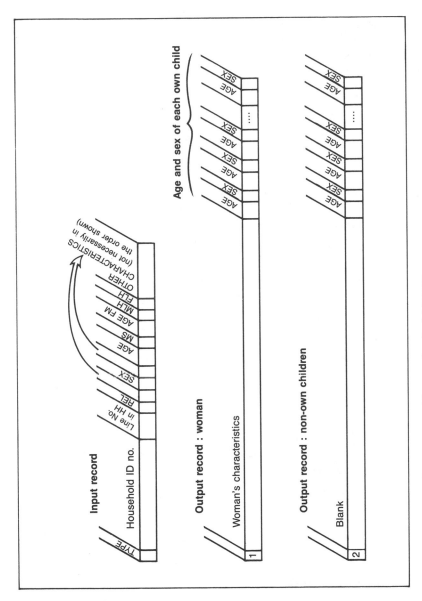

Figure C.1. Input and output record layouts for the MATCH program

Note: HH denotes household; REL, relationship to household head; MS, marital status; AGE FM, age at first marriage; MLH, number of male children living in the household (for a particular woman); FLH, number of female children living in the household.

TAB

The second-stage tabulation program, TAB, takes the output from MATCH and creates the own-children matrix. In this matrix, matched (own) children are tabulated by child's age and mother's age. The matrix includes a tabulation of numbers of women by woman's age and a tabulation of number of children by child's age. If the Brass method (Brass 1975) of estimating child mortality is to be used, the number of children ever born to women by woman's age and the number of children still living (or surviving) by woman's age are tabulated as well. Listing C.2 presents an example of the basic tabulation program, and an example of the resulting output table is shown in Table C.1. The program is also written in PL/I.

Listing C.2. TAB

```
00010   TAB:
00020        PROCEDURE OPTIONS(MAIN);
00030
00040        DCL   OWA(1,15:67,-4:15) FLOAT,
00050              NAM(1) CHAR(8) INIT('TOTAL    ');
00060
00070        DCL INFILE RECORD INPUT SEQUENTIAL BUFFERED
00080            ENV(CONSECUTIVE FB RECSIZE(137) BLKSIZE(13700) TOTAL),
00090
00100            INAREA CHAR(137),
00110          1 WOMAN DEF INAREA,
00120            2 TYPE    CHAR(1),
00130            2 REL     CHAR(1),
00140            2 FIL1    CHAR(11),
00150            2 AGE     PIC'99',
00160            2 EDUC    CHAR(6),
00170            2 CEB     PIC'99',
00180            2 CLWM    PIC'99',
00190            2 INFFACTOR   PIC'9999',
00200            2 FILL7   CHAR(1),
00210            2 MARIT   CHAR(1),
00220            2 KIDREL  CHAR(1),
00230            2 KIDD(15),
00240              3 SEX CHAR(1),   3 CAGE PIC'99',
00250              3   INFFAC PIC'9999',
00260          1 NONOWN DEF INAREA,
00270            2 FIL5   CHAR(12),
00280            2 NKID(17),
00290              3 KSEX CHAR(1),   3 NAGE PIC '99',
00300              3 INF PIC'9999';
00310
00320
00330        OWA = 0;
00340        ON ENDFILE(INFILE) GO TO PAU;
00350
00360   NEXT:
00370        READ FILE(INFILE) INTO (INAREA);
00380        CALL FILLG;
00390        GO TO NEXT;
00400   PAU:
00410        IA = 1;
00420        CALL OUTIT (    IA,NAM(IA));
00430  1FILLG:
00440        PROCEDURE;
```

Listing C.2. TAB *(continued)*

```
00450        IA = 1;
00460        IF TYPE='1' THEN DO;
00470           JAG = AGE;
00480   /*
00490           COUNT NO OF WOMEN     */
00500           OWA(IA,JAG,-3) = OWA(IA,JAG,-3)  + INFFACTOR;
00510   /*
00520           GET CEB, CSURV, CURRENT MARRIED */
00530          CSURV = CLWM;
00540        IF CEB > 20 THEN CEB = 0;
00550        IF CSURV > 20 THEN CSURV = 0 ;
00560           OWA(IA,JAG,-2)  =  OWA(IA,JAG,-2) + CEB * INFFACTOR;
00570           OWA(IA,JAG,-1)  =  OWA(IA,JAG,-1) + CSURV * INFFACTOR;
00580
00590           IF MARIT= '2' THEN DO; OWA(IA,JAG,-4) = OWA(IA,JAG,-4)+
00600                                    INFFACTOR;
00610                            END;
00620   /*
00630   NOW TALLY CHILDREN   */
00640           DO   I= 1 TO 15;
00650           IF SEX(I) = ' ' THEN RETURN;
00660           KA = CAGE(I);
00670           OWA(IA,JAG,KA) = OWA(IA,JAG,KA) + INFFAC (I);
00680           END;
00690           END;
00700   /*
00710   HANDLE NON-OWN   */
00720        ELSE DO   I= 1 TO 17;
00730                IF KSEX(I) = ' ' THEN RETURN;
00740                KA = NAGE(I) ;
00750                OWA(IA,67,KA) = OWA(IA,67,KA) + INF (I);
00760                END;
00770        END FILLG;
00780 1OUTIT:
00790        PROCEDURE   (IA,NAMD);
00800
00810        DCL  NAMD CHAR(8), IA FIXED BIN;
00820
00830        OWA(IA,66,*) = 0;    OWA(IA,67,-1) = 0;
00840   /*
00850   GET  COLUMN TOTALS        */
00860        DO J= 15 TO 65;
00870        OWA(IA,66,*) =  OWA(IA,66,*) + OWA(IA,J,*);
00880        END;
00890        DO J = 0 TO 14;
00900        OWA (IA,67,-1) = OWA(IA,67,-1) + OWA(IA,67,J);
00910        END;
00920   /*
00930   NOW  PRINTIT   */
00940        PUT PAGE EDIT (' AREA IS ', NAMD) (A,A(8));
00950        PUT SKIP(2) EDIT
00960           ('AGE') (A)
00970           ('TOTAL'      ,'CEB',  'CSURV',(I DO I=0 TO 14))
00980           (X(3), COL(6), A, COL(17), A, COL(23), A, 15 F(7));
00990        DO I = 15 TO 65;
01000        PUT SKIP EDIT (I,(OWA(IA,I,K) DO K= -3 TO 14))
01010                      (F(2), F(9), 2 F(8), 15 F(7));
01020        END;
01030        PUT SKIP EDIT ('TOT',(OWA(IA,66,K) DO K=-3 TO 14))
01040                      (A, F(8), 2 F(8), 15 F(7));
01050        PUT SKIP EDIT (OWA(IA,67,-1),'NON-OWN-DATA',
01060                      (OWA(IA,67,K) DO K=0 TO 14))
01070                      (X(3),F(6),X(3),A,X(3),15 F(7));
01080        END OUTIT;
01090        END FSTG2;
```

Table C.1. Output from the TAB program

Women's age	Total women	CEB	CS	<1	1	2	3	4
10	1,808,478	0	0	0	0	0	0	0
11	1,443,242	0	0	0	0	0	0	0
12	1,675,303	0	0	0	0	0	0	0
13	1,467,245	2,082	1,998	1,764	0	0	0	0
14	1,360,339	8,728	6,664	3,065	2,050	0	0	0
15	1,502,946	26,046	23,640	12,865	6,422	3,405	0	326
16	1,290,305	94,582	82,194	43,680	18,425	7,159	4,184	2,257
17	1,412,854	240,076	195,477	91,885	52,866	20,165	14,077	3,511
18	1,391,103	459,748	403,720	169,718	98,040	64,654	33,254	13,319
19	1,260,466	772,858	667,969	214,240	160,997	107,231	76,729	38,029
20	1,543,351	1,253,931	1,096,794	293,714	247,525	171,899	145,695	104,795
21	913,132	914,269	812,304	170,728	159,543	146,737	120,414	77,341
22	886,601	1,184,030	1,029,443	199,112	169,328	156,638	151,267	111,924
23	778,839	1,258,633	1,090,795	197,422	152,623	150,522	142,599	125,731
24	925,528	1,803,499	1,538,394	196,894	192,088	189,342	194,406	175,591
25	1,478,282	3,267,498	2,766,261	284,867	328,658	305,821	330,684	322,490
26	712,747	1,769,840	1,530,626	146,159	154,125	159,637	172,555	160,798
27	765,977	2,136,495	1,817,079	157,604	152,519	173,365	171,442	173,467
28	630,875	1,965,838	1,674,515	106,281	131,925	130,876	145,072	154,047
29	809,879	2,805,178	2,362,673	143,857	161,281	182,077	176,092	187,352
30	1,423,895	5,314,087	4,344,995	247,008	245,365	259,839	311,106	332,889
31	534,518	2,099,852	1,752,258	90,275	92,757	123,662	111,667	115,555
32	664,162	2,751,039	2,264,790	112,810	110,476	107,336	131,692	133,973
33	565,786	2,494,632	2,095,985	85,205	96,091	92,103	121,768	124,513
34	833,899	3,730,699	3,102,768	102,534	146,377	133,404	161,338	161,159
35	1,513,382	7,288,969	5,775,276	173,929	182,414	222,392	255,388	292,818
36	632,264	3,196,804	2,588,639	67,969	88,789	80,165	109,981	122,104
37	627,941	3,189,765	2,529,081	59,881	68,253	79,060	106,950	109,287
38	562,033	3,036,943	2,414,122	46,690	64,228	78,956	93,796	103,387
39	817,327	4,219,270	3,379,926	58,387	66,485	78,999	105,780	119,396
40	1,298,898	6,588,296	5,042,915	63,349	80,373	97,918	118,339	157,619
41	473,904	2,471,041	1,945,309	27,849	30,266	37,483	55,278	58,330
42	469,143	2,577,798	1,971,697	24,150	23,942	32,177	45,611	57,917
43	399,854	2,346,646	1,770,392	15,381	25,489	25,527	28,527	45,968
44	536,008	2,776,095	2,125,204	21,599	23,856	27,725	37,769	45,609
45	1,077,221	5,552,327	4,129,881	19,284	2,2501	44,084	60,408	78,840
46	373,704	2,076,555	1,517,096	4,897	9,304	7,570	17,561	22,098
47	373,568	2,108,587	1,593,502	3,731	8,376	12,851	17,424	19,119
48	360,411	1,966,408	1,418,990	2,929	8,601	8,203	13,805	22,035
49	495,081	2,431,552	1,806,642	8,586	8,238	8,176	15,328	17,106
50	815,176	4,097,908	2,832,837	0	4,142	6,850	9,681	14,173
51	367,306	1,963,227	1,402,291	0	0	3,047	4,047	11,050
52	348,913	1,813,132	1,302,363	0	0	0	3,015	3,629
53	250,904	1,226,910	893,167	0	0	0	0	3,402
54	361,211	1,759,624	1,269,730	0	0	0	0	0
55	668,496	3,096,172	2,176,559	0	0	0	0	0
56	193,103	966,421	690,525	0	0	0	0	0
57	177,559	858,214	609,962	0	0	0	0	0
58	168,595	845,432	580,261	0	0	0	0	0
59	311,994	1,412,746	984,814	0	0	0	0	0
60	667,097	3,074,600	2,106,788	0	0	0	0	0
61	144,584	666,250	478,823	0	0	0	0	0
62	138,673	684,383	463,874	0	0	0	0	0
63	115,014	586,927	412,162	0	0	0	0	0
64	173,661	780,985	534,734	0	0	0	0	0
65	357,058	1,661,604	1,104,588	0	0	0	0	0
Non-own children				34,782	55,452	89,419	157,446	151,895

CEB—number of children ever born.
CS—number of children surviving.

Children's age

5	6	7	8	9	10	11	12	13	14
0	0	0	0	0	0	0	0	0	0
0	0	0	0	0	0	0	0	0	0
0	0	0	0	0	0	0	0	0	0
0	0	0	0	0	0	0	0	0	0
0	0	0	0	0	0	0	0	0	0
0	0	0	0	0	0	0	0	0	0
0	0	0	0	0	0	0	0	0	0
1,201	764	0	0	0	0	0	0	0	0
2,783	344	0	0	0	0	0	0	0	0
20,278	5,296	5,382	1,905	0	0	0	0	0	0
44,845	22,728	15,965	5,562	161	0	0	0	0	0
39,701	25,310	15,648	4,440	2,449	1,850	0	0	0	0
80,490	43,021	22,521	14,610	4,233	4,585	1,626	0	0	0
105,453	74,789	37,604	25,409	9,703	6,978	2,675	1,518	0	0
130,431	124,914	84,011	49,889	33,688	23,741	9,958	8,140	2,231	0
250,272	225,435	201,761	125,469	78,667	82,495	32,868	25,421	11,463	7,906
147,470	138,032	108,567	88,301	58,634	49,831	28,729	16,888	6,676	2,420
150,792	138,224	155,650	112,851	96,432	89,402	61,842	34,775	14,383	7,285
152,704	139,217	124,830	128,478	93,715	105,102	50,584	53,790	25,223	10,531
179,598	181,486	184,109	138,667	160,319	117,009	106,046	78,707	60,506	48,476
330,772	306,812	329,673	301,294	271,628	276,306	186,711	209,477	121,224	88,583
133,716	133,536	114,950	113,281	99,524	109,572	92,441	86,524	59,189	44,314
168,406	138,874	161,226	131,766	137,327	141,815	114,520	118,509	103,609	77,664
129,899	126,288	125,297	142,939	112,170	133,746	115,201	110,426	97,697	85,861
171,532	173,807	186,544	159,667	179,565	158,759	164,778	145,936	130,208	140,517
306,958	308,752	315,135	332,791	300,169	354,156	263,894	338,532	266,702	228,212
135,890	127,590	137,694	139,037	138,704	146,200	125,469	142,634	118,144	114,267
124,310	111,057	139,031	121,795	128,967	129,081	120,330	128,016	113,151	108,949
108,750	113,101	117,807	122,868	121,813	129,600	101,641	131,641	100,546	95,365
124,522	137,402	132,706	134,005	154,528	152,917	138,552	167,255	147,020	137,131
172,928	196,325	213,564	210,093	211,315	259,370	170,947	257,526	232,571	199,439
54,551	69,744	73,135	71,196	84,335	76,168	84,910	90,840	91,548	81,584
66,924	55,916	71,341	82,776	77,409	89,414	78,738	85,633	83,724	82,751
44,296	61,319	57,515	60,360	70,304	69,021	70,601	90,903	72,774	68,071
49,340	66,587	64,662	61,533	83,982	57,627	80,393	80,530	81,425	95,250
71,105	106,612	110,022	126,354	130,025	134,202	139,585	170,384	159,676	145,013
36,600	33,883	34,481	47,262	45,734	64,533	44,264	56,605	53,827	57,949
25,348	27,347	40,919	41,692	47,825	59,068	46,784	56,036	63,949	67,863
19,507	22,500	32,912	33,789	39,543	38,954	50,178	54,304	53,443	50,159
21,524	19,740	29,932	22,079	37,256	68,096	41,284	47,488	51,739	58,200
21,124	27,706	42,463	38,546	38,297	68,096	41,284	75,964	74,933	72,895
6,987	10,334	12,976	17,668	27,886	32,709	25,114	41,905	38,664	33,885
4,481	7,142	8,069	19,125	20,756	24,817	15,558	33,134	25,208	32,260
3,432	6,548	11,385	5,682	10,645	18,321	13,272	21,796	23,353	17,976
5,753	10,658	11,990	9,748	17,390	15,086	17,855	34,639	26,037	33,810
0	9,285	7,697	11,557	13,084	26,262	24,210	36,456	43,873	38,078
0	0	4,482	4,762	4,766	7,379	8,108	6,332	6,123	11,889
0	0	0	3,927	3,413	6,117	3,030	9,917	4,079	11,487
0	0	0	0	614	3,948	3,849	3,734	6,904	7,765
0	0	0	0	0	2,524	750	11,518	4,960	13,121
0	0	0	0	0	0	3,450	12,931	13,169	9,891
0	0	0	0	0	0	0	3,286	2,100	2,772
0	0	0	0	0	0	0	0	275	3,129
0	0	0	0	0	0	0	0	0	2,311
0	0	0	0	0	0	0	0	0	0
0	0	0	0	0	0	0	0	0	0
166,076	199,214	278,252	257,022	267,090	335,016	283,350	407,849	379,340	389,144

If mother's line number is used and coded in the census, stages 1 and 2 are easily combined. An example of a PL/I program, MATCHTAB, for the combined match and tabulation is also given (Listing C.3). For the processing of census data most national statistical offices are equipped with elaborate tabulation programs that can produce tables for the whole country as well as for subpopulations in a single step. At the East–West Population Institute, the own-children tabulation programs have been developed using two well-known tabulation programs, COCENTS and TPL. These programs, which are alternatives to the PL/I program presented here, are also available to interested users upon request.

Listing C.3. MATCHTAB

```
00010    MATCHTAB:PROC OPTIONS(MAIN);
00020    DCL INDO FILE RECORD SEQUENTIAL BUFFERED INPUT
00030         ENV(CONSECUTIVE FB RECSIZE(160) BLKSIZE(12000) TOTAL),
00040         (STAGE2,DISK) FILE STREAM OUTPUT,
00050         PRIN FILE PRINT;
00060    DCL HHM(35,9) DECIMAL FIXED(4) INIT((315) 0),
00070         (ISLE(58,18,3),P(58,18,3)) FIXED BIN(31,0) INIT((3132) 0),
00080         JX FIXED DEC(2) INIT(0),
00090         YOUNG_MOM(0:9) FIXED BINARY INIT((10) 0),
00100         XPROV CHAR(2),
00110         MAJ_ISLE CHAR(13),
00120         XHHNO DEC FIXED(3) INIT(0),
00130         XAREA FIXED DEC(1),
00140         XMOM(25) BIN FIXED(15,0) INIT((25) 0),
00150         AREA(3) CHAR(5) INIT('URBAN','RURAL','TOTAL');
00160    DCL REC CHAR(160),
00170    UR    PIC'9'    DEF REC POS(14),      /* URBAN/RURAL         */
00180    PNO   PIC'99'   DEF REC POS(25),      /* PERSON'S LINE NO.   */
00190    SEX   PIC'9'    DEF REC POS(27),      /* SEX                 */
00200    AGE   PIC'99'   DEF REC POS(33),      /* AGE                 */
00210    MA_ST PIC'9'    DEF REC POS(42),      /* MOTHER'S STATUS     */
00220    MA_NO PIC'99'   DEF REC POS(43),      /* MOTHER'S LINE NO.   */
00230    CEB   PIC'99'   DEF REC POS(101),     /* CHILDREN EVER BORN  */
00240    CLH   PIC'99'   DEF REC POS(103),     /* CHILDREN AT HOME    */
00250    CLA   PIC'99'   DEF REC POS(105),     /* CHILDREN AWAY       */
00260    INFL  PIC'9999' DEF REC POS(154),     /* INFLATION FACTOR    */
00270    PROV  CHAR(2)   DEF REC POS(159);     /* PROVINCE NO.        */
00280    OPEN  FILE(PRIN) OUTPUT PAGESIZE(67);
00290    /*
00300     READ IN MAJOR ISLAND NAME & FIRST PROVINCE CODE
00310                                                         */
00320    GET EDIT(MAJ_ISLE,XPROV) (A(13),A(2));
00330    ON ENDFILE(INDO) BEGIN;
00340         CALL ADD_PROV;
00350         CALL OUT_AREA(P, 1);
00360         CALL MOM_ERR;
00370         CALL OUT_AREA(ISLE, 2);
00380         GO TO EOJ;
00390         END;
00400
00410     RR: READ FILE(INDO) INTO(REC);
00420
00430        IF PROV ~= XPROV THEN DO;       /* NEW PROVINCE */
00440                CALL ADD_PROV;          /* OLD PROVONCE TOTALS */
00450                CALL OUT_AREA(P, 1); /* PRINT PROVINCE MATRIX */
00460                CALL MOM_ERR;
00470                CALL INIT;       /* INITIALIZE PROVINCE VARIABLES */
00480                END;
00490
```

Listing C.3. MATCHTAB *(continued)*

```
00500        IF PNO < 77 THEN CALL HH_ARRAY;      /* PERSON RECORD        */
00510          ELSE IF PNO = 77 THEN GO TO RR;    /* MORTALITY RECORD     */
00520          ELSE CALL TALLY;                   /* HOUSEHOLD RECORD     */
00530
00540    GO TO RR;
00550    HH_ARRAY: PROC;
00560    /*
00570        THIS PROCEDURE INCREMENTS THE HOUSEHOLD PERSON COUNTER & STORES
00580        SELECTED CHARACTERISTICS FROM THAT PERSON RECORD INTO THE ARRAY
00590        HHM
00600                                                                    */
00610
00620        JX = JX + 1;
00630        IF JX = 1 THEN XAREA = UR;
00640        HHM(JX,1) = SEX;
00650        HHM(JX,2) = AGE;
00660        HHM(JX,3) = MA_ST;
00670        HHM(JX,4) = MA_NO;
00680        HHM(JX,5) = INFL;
00690        HHM(JX,6) = PNO;
00700        HHM(JX,7) = CEB;
00710        HHM(JX,8) = CLH;
00720        HHM(JX,9) = CLA;
00730    END HH_ARRAY;
00740    TALLY: PROCEDURE;
00750    /*
00760       THIS PROCEDURE CHECKS EACH HOUSEHOLD MEMBER AND DOES THE FOLLOWING:
00770       1. TABULATES WOMEN DATA.
00780
00790          WOMEN AGED 10-65 ARE TABULATED BY AGE, CEB, CLH & CLA.  IF CEB,
00800          CLH & CLA < 30. INFLATION FACTOR (WGT) IS USED.
00810
00820
00830       2. TABULATES MOTHER-CHILD MATRIX.
00840
00850          IF A PERSON'S AGE IS 0-14, THIS PERSON IS CONSIDERED A CHILD.
00860          IF ITS MOTHER IS PRESENT, THE HOUSEHOLD ARRAY(HHM) IS SEARCHED
00870          FOR THE HOUSEHOLD MEMBER WHOSE LINE NO. MATCHES THE MOTHER'S
00880          LINE NO. INDICATED ON THE CHILD'S RECORD.
00890
00900          IF THE MOTHER'S LINE NO. IS > JX (THE TOTAL NO. OF PERSONS IN
00910          THE HOUSEHOLD) OR = 0 OR = 99 (CODES FOR UNKNOWN) THE CHILD
00920          IS NON-OWN.
00930
00940          IF THE MOTHER'S PRESENT AGE IS <10 OR >65 THE CHILD IS NON-OWN.
00950
00960          IF THE MOTHER'S AGE AT THE BIRTH OF THE CHILD HAD BEEN 11-49,
00970          THE CHILD IS AN OWN CHILD.  OTHERWISE, THE CHILD IS NON-OWN &
00980          ITS MOTHER IS TABULATED BY HER AGE AT THE BIRTH OF THE CHILD.
00990    */
01000    DCL (JAGE, MOM_AGE, MOM_LNO, AGE_AT_BIRTH, INDX) FIXED DEC(2),
01010        WGT FIXED DEC(4);
01020
01030    DO K=1 TO JX;      /* JX=TOTAL NO. OF PERSONS IN THIS HOUSEHOLD */
01040
01050    JAGE=HHM(K, 2);
01060     WGT=HHM(K, 5);
01070
01080    IF HHM(K,1)=2 & (JAGE>9 & JAGE<66) & HHM(K,7)<30 & HHM(K,8)<30 &
01090        HHM(K,9)<30 THEN DO;    /* TABULATE WOMEN DATA */
01100
01110        P(JAGE-7,1,XAREA) = P(JAGE-7,1,XAREA) + WGT;
01120        P(JAGE-7,2,XAREA) = P(JAGE-7,2,XAREA) + HHM(K,7)*WGT;
01130        P(JAGE-7,3,XAREA) = P(JAGE-7,3,XAREA) + (HHM(K,8) + HHM(K,9))*WGT;
01140
01150        END;
```

Listing C.3. MATCHTAB *(continued)*

```
01160
01170    IF JAGE>14 THEN GO TO NEXT_PERSON;    /* CHECK FOR CHILD */
01180
01190    MOM_PRESENT: IF HHM(K,3)=1 THEN DO;   /* CHECK FOR MOTHER STATUS */
01200    MOM_LNO=HHM(K,4);
01210
01220    FIND_MOM: DO L=1 TO JX;
01230       IF MOM_LNO=HHM(L,6) THEN DO;   /* MOTHER FOUND            */
01240
01250          MOM_AGE=HHM(L,2);              /* MOTHER'S PRESENT AGE  */
01260          IF MOM_AGE>65 THEN GO TO NOWN;
01270
01280          IF MOM_AGE<10 THEN DO;
01290             YOUNG_MOM(MOM_AGE)=YOUNG_MOM(MOM_AGE) + 1;
01300             GO TO NOWN;
01310             END;
01320
01330          AGE_AT_BIRTH=MOM_AGE - JAGE; /* MOTHER'S AGE AT BIRTH OF CHILD
01340
01350          IF AGE_AT_BIRTH>10 & AGE_AT_BIRTH<50 THEN DO;   /* OWN CHILD */
01360             P(MOM_AGE-7,JAGE+4,XAREA) = P(MOM_AGE-7,JAGE+4,XAREA) + WGT;
01370             GO TO NEXT_PERSON;
01380             END;
01390
01400          ELSE DO;
01410             IF AGE_AT_BIRTH>0 * AGE_AT_BIRTH<11 THEN INDX=AGE_AT_BIRTH;
01420                ELSE IF AGE_AT_BIRTH>49 & AGE_AT_BIRTH<65 THEN
01430                   INDX=AGE_AT_BIRTH - 39;
01440                ELSE GO TO NOWN;
01450             XMOM(INDX)=XMOM(INDX) +1;
01460             GO TO NOWN;
01470             END;
01480          END;
01490
01500       END FIND_MOM;
01510
01520    END;   /* END MOM_PRESENT GROUP  */
01530
01540    NOWN: P(1,JAGE+4,XAREA) = P(1,JAGE+4,XAREA) + WGT;  /* NON-OWN CHILD
01550
01560    NEXT_PERSON: END;
01570
01580
01590    HHM=0;          /* RE-INITIALIZE HOUSEHOLD ARRAY, PERSON COUNTER */
01600    JX=0;
01610
01620    END TALLY;
01630    ADD_PROV:  PROC;
01640    /*
01650       THIS PROCEDURE COMPUTES THE TOTAL LINE FOR WOMEN & CHILDREN
01660       AND ADDS URBAN AND RURAL TO GET TOTAL PROVINCE.
01670                                                                   */
01680          DO I= 3 TO 58;
01690          P(2,*,*) = P(2,*,*) + P(I,*,*);
01700          END;
01710    /*
01720          SUM URBAN & RURAL AREAS OF PROVINCE TO GET TOTAL PROVINCE
01730                                                                   */
01740             P(*,*,3) = P(*,*,3) + P(*,*,1) + P(*,*,2);
01750             ISLE(*,*,*) = ISLE(*,*,*) + P(*,*,*);
01760
01770    END ADD_PROV;
01780    OUT_AREA: PROC(X,TYPE);
01790    /*
01800       THIS PROCEDURE WRITES THE MOTHER-CHILD MATRIX TO A PRINT FILE.
```

Listing C.3. MATCHTAB *(continued)*

```
01810    & TO A TAPE FILE FOR INPUT TO STAGE 3 OF THE OWN CHILDREN PACKAGE.
01820
01830    IF THE AREA IS A MAJOR ISLAND (I.E. TYPE=2), THE MATRIX IS WRITTEN
01840    TO A DISK FILE FOR COMPUTATION OF THE MOTHER-CHILD MATRIX FOR TOTAL
01850    INDONESIA.
01860
01870                                                                        *
01880    DCL X(*,*,*) FIXED BIN(31,0),
01890        NAME CHAR(13) INIT((13) ' '),
01900        TYPE FIXED BIN,       /* 1=PROVINCE    2=MAJOR ISLANDS    */
01910        TITLE(6) CHAR(132) VARYING INIT(
01920    'OWN CHILDREN ANALYSIS BASED ON 1976 INDONESIA INTERCENSAL SURVEY - PHA
01930    SE II: MOTHER-CHILD MATRIX',
01940    (132) '-',
01950    ' AGE',
01960    ' OF    TOTAL',
01970    'A G E   O F   C H I L D',
01980    'WOMEN WOMEN    CEB        CS      < 1      1      2      3      4      5
01990         6      7       8        9      10     11     12     13     14');
02000
02010    DO K=1 TO 3;    /* URBAN/RURAL/TOTAL  */
02020
02030    IF X(2,1,K)=0 THEN GO TO NEXT_AREA; /* TEST FOR ALL URBAL/RURAL AREA */
02040
02050    /* PRINT HEADINGS, NON-OWN CHILDREN & TOTALS LINE    */
02060
02070    IF TYPE=1 THEN NAME='PROVINCE '  || XPROV;
02080        ELSE NAME=MAJ_ISLE;
02090
02100    PUT FILE(PRIN) EDIT
02110        (TITLE(1),NAME,AREA(K), (TITLE(N) DO N=2 TO 6), TITLE(2),
02120        'NON',(X(1,J,K) DO J=4 TO 18),
02130        'TOT',   (X(2,J,K) DO J=1 TO 18) )
02140      (PAGE, COL(1), A, COL(113), A, COL(128), A,
02150       SKIP(0), COL(1), A, COL(1), A, COL(1), A,
02160       SKIP(0), COL(71), A, COL(1), A, SKIP(0), COL(1), A,
02170       SKIP(2), COL(1), A, COL(28), 15 F(7),
02180       COL(1), A, 3 F(8), 15 F(7) );
02190    /*
02200        WRITE NON-OWN LINE TO TAPE. OMIT TOTALS LINE.
02210        IF MAJOR ISLAND, WRITE DISK FILE
02220    */
02230    PUT FILE(STAGE2) EDIT(NAME,AREA(K), (X(1,J,K) DO J=4 TO 18))
02240       ( COL(1), A, X(1), A, SKIP, COL(23), 15 F(7) );
02250
02260    IF TYPE=2 THEN
02270     PUT FILE(DISK) EDIT(NAME, AREA(K), (X(1,J,K) DO J = 4 TO 18))
02280                       (COL(1), A, X(1), A, SKIP, COL(23), 15 F(7));
02290    /*
02300      WRITE REST OF MATRIX
02310    */
02320    DO I=3 TO 58;
02330     PUT FILE(PRIN) EDIT(I+7,  (X(I,J,K) DO J=1 TO 18))
02340        (COL(1),F(2),X(1), 3 F(8), 15 F(7));
02350
02360     PUT FILE(STAGE2) EDIT((X(I,J,K) DO J=1 TO 18))
02370        (COL(1), 3 F(8), 15 F(7));
02380
02390     IF TYPE=2 THEN PUT FILE(DISK) EDIT((X(I,J,K) DO J=1 TO 18))
02400        (COL(1), 3 F(8), 15 F(7) );
02410
02420    END;
02430
02440    NEXT_AREA: END;
02450
```

Listing C.3. MATCHTAB *(continued)*

```
02460
02470    END OUT_AREA;
02480    MOM_ERR: PROC;
02490    /*
02500        PRINT FREQUENCY DISTRIBUTION OF MOTHERS EXCLUDED FROM
02510        WOMAN-CHILD MATRIX DUE TO INELIGIBLE AGE AT BIRTH OF CHILD
02520                                                                    */
02530      PUT FILE(PRIN)
02540          EDIT('FREQUENCY DISTRIBUTION OF MOTHERS AGED 1 - 10 & 50-64 A
02550    RTH OF CHILD', 'PROVINCE ', XPROV,
02560            '    1    2    3    4    5    6    7    8    9   10   50   51
02570    2   53   54   55   56   57   58   59   60   61   62   63   64',
02580          (XMOM(J) DO J=1 TO 25))
02590            (PAGE,COL(1), A, COL(1), A, A, SKIP(2), COL(1), A, SKIP(3),
02600             COL(1), 25 F(5));
02610
02620
02630    /*
02640      PRINT FREQUENCY DISTRIBUTION OF MOTHERS WHOSE PRESENT AGE IS < 10
02650
02660
02670    PUT FILE(PRIN)
02680        EDIT('FREQUENCY DISTRIBUTION OF MOTHERS WHOSE PRESENTAGE IS 0 - 9
02690    (L DO L=0 TO 9 ), (YOUNG_MOM(L) DO L=0 TO 9))
02700    (SKIP(4), COL(1), A, SKIP(2), COL(1), 10 F(5), SKIP(3),
02710          COL(1), 10 F(5));
02720
02730    END MOM_ERR;
02740    INIT:  PROC;
02750    /*
02760      RESET PROVINCE WOMAN-CHILD ARRAY TO ZERO.
02770      RESET YOUNG(YOUNG_MOM) & YOUNG-OLD(XMOM) MOTHER COUNTERS TO ZERO.
02780      ASSIGN NEW PROVINCE CODE
02790
02800      P = 0;
02810      HHM = 0;
02820      JX = 0;
02830      YOUNG_MOM = 0;
02840      XMOM = 0;
02850      XPROV = PROV;
02860
02870    END INIT;
02880    EOJ: END OWNC;
```

OWCH3

The third-stage programs, collectively called OWCH3, take the own-children table generated by TAB and compute age-specific birth rates and related measures. In addition to the core subroutine OWN that does the reverse survival and adjusts for unmatched children and enumeration errors, optional subroutines are available to estimate mortality using the Brass method, to compute regional model life tables, to interpolate abridged life tables, and to compute survival ratios. Among them, only the subroutine for the last of these, SURVIV, is listed in this appendix; the other subroutines may be obtained upon request. (For historical reasons the SURVIV subroutine yields forward-survival ratios rather than reverse-survival ratios. The forward-survival ratios are inverted to reverse-survival ratios in the OWN subroutine.)

Control flow. The MAIN program of the third stage (Listing C.4) determines the order of execution of these subroutines as specified by the user, generates headings for output, and performs other bookkeeping operations. The program is written in FORTRAN. Figure C.2 shows alternative paths of the program flow depending on the user's selection. The output generated by this program has already been illustrated in Chapter 7.

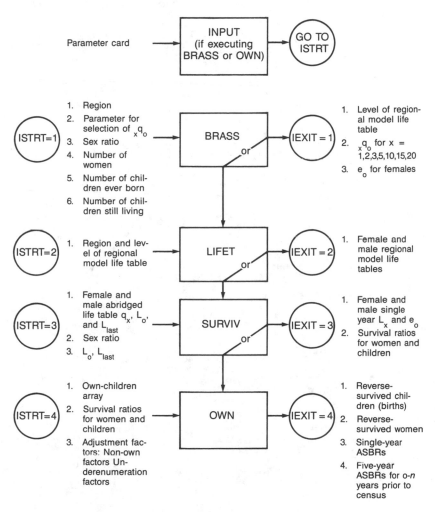

Figure C.2. Schematic of control flow in MAIN program

Listing C.4. MAIN

```
00010 C
00020 C
00030 C      MAIN
00040 C      OWNCH3 - OWN CHILDREN STAGE 3
00050 C      EAST-WEST POPULATION INSTITUTE
00060 C      EAST-WEST CENTER
00070 C      HONOLULU, HAWAII
00080 C
00090 C
00100 C
00110 C                      LAST DAY OF REVISION -- JULY 20, 1979
00120 C
00130        DIMENSION TAB(16,51),WMN(51),CS(51),CEB(51),AREA(50),ARAMRT(50)
00140      1 ARA(10),TITL(100),TILMRT(100),TBNO(2),TBMRT(2),STRD(7,2),
00150      2 ENUM(15),ENUMW(51),UNK(15),SR(16,52),COMNT(20),NNEG(15)
00160        INTEGER*4 SELEC,SUMARY(2,10)
00170        INTEGER*4 POPID(5),UPPER,QSELEC,REGLAB(4)
00180        REAL*4 LEVEL(15),LIFTBF(18,15),LIFTBM(18,15),NQO(231),NOWN(15),
00190      1NW(7),NCEB(7),NCS(7),LLVEL,LLXF(15),LLXM(15),LLXFO(15),LLXMO(15
00200        EQUIVALENCE (ARA(1),AREA(1))
00210        DATA REGLAB/'W','N','E','S' /
00220 C
00230 C
00240 C
00250 C      READ IN PARAMETERS
00260 C
00270   100 CONTINUE
00280        MRTFLG=0
00290        READ(5,10,END=999) ISTRT,IEXIT,QSELEC,NREG,LOAGE,IPCH,ITP2,IPRII
00300      1 ITP3,IPRIN3,ITP4,LP,NYEAR,SEXRAT
00310        PRINT 15,ISTRT,IEXIT,QSELEC,NREG,LOAGE,IPCH,ITP2,IPRIN2,ITP3,
00320      1        IPRIN3,ITP4,LP,NYEAR,SEXRAT
00330        IF (ITP4.EQ.0) ITP4=6
00340        IF (IEXIT .EQ. 0) IEXIT= 4
00350        IF (IEXIT.NE.4) GO TO 55
00360        READ(5,50,END=990) IYEAR,MON,SUMARY,ENUM,ENUMW, NOWN,STRD,POPID
00370        PRINT 70,IYEAR,MON,ENUM,ENUMW,STRD,POPID
00380        IF (ITP4.NE.6) WRITE(ITP4,70) IYEAR,MON,ENUM,ENUMW,STRD,POPID
00390        DO 56 I=1,5
00400        READ(5,80) COMNT
00410        PRINT 85, COMNT
00420    56 IF (ITP4.NE.6) WRITE(ITP4,85) COMNT
00430 C
00440 C      INITIALIZE FOR DEFAULTS
00450 C
00460    55 CONTINUE
00470        IF(MON.LT.7) IYEAR=IYEAR-1
00480        IFIT=0
00490        IERR=1
00500        IF (ITP2.EQ.4.OR.ITP3.EQ.4.OR.ITP4.EQ.4) GO TO 996
00510        IF (ITP2.EQ.8.OR.ITP3.EQ.8.OR.ITP4.EQ.8) GO TO 996
00520        IF (ISTRT.EQ.0) ISTRT=1
00530        IF (IEXIT.EQ.0) IEXIT=4
00540        IF (QSELEC.EQ.0) QSELEC=4
00550        IF (NREG.EQ.0) NREG=1
00560        IF (LOAGE.EQ.0) LOAGE = 15
00570        IF (LOAGE.LT.15.OR.LOAGE.GT.30) GO TO 995
00580        IF (SEXRAT.EQ.0) SEXRAT=1.05
00590        IF (NYEAR.EQ.0) NYEAR=15
00600        IF (LP.EQ.0) LP=1
00610        MRTID = REGLAB(NREG)
00620        IF (ISTRT.LT.1.OR.IEXIT.GT.4) GO TO 980
00630 C
00640 C
```

Listing C.4. MAIN *(continued)*

```
00650 C      ABEND IF EXIT POINT PRECEEDS ENTRY POINT
00660        IF(ISTRT-IEXIT) 800,800,991
00670    800 CONTINUE
00680        DO 700 LOOP=1,LP
00690        IF (ISTRT.GT.1.AND.IEXIT.LT.4) GO TO (1,2,3,4),ISTRT
00700 C
00710 C
00720 C      READ IN WOMEN, CHILDREN-EVER-BORN,CHILDREN-SURVIVING
00730        CALL INPUT (IFLAG,NOWN,NROW,NCOL,TITL,AREA,TBNO,WMN,CEB,CS,TAB)
00740 C      ON ENDFILE INPUT GO TO END
00750        IF (IFLAG-8) 106,997,999
00760 C
00770    106 UPPER = NROW + 14
00780        IUP= UPPER -13
00790        IUPC = NCOL - 2
00800        ILO1 = LOAGE - 14
00810        IF ((MRTFLG.NE.0).AND.(ISTRT.NE.1))  GO TO 5
00820        IF (ISTRT.NE.1) GO TO 200
00830        DO 110 J=1,7
00840        NW(J)=0.0
00850        NCEB(J)=0.0
00860        NCS(J) = 0.0
00870        SUM = 0
00880        ILO2=ILO1+4
00890        DO 105 I=ILO1,ILO2
00900        NW(J)=NW(J)+WMN(I)
00910        NCEB(J)=NCEB(J)+CEB(I)
00920    105 NCS(J)=NCS(J) + CS(I)
00930    110 ILO1=ILO2+1
00940    200 GO TO (1,2,3,4),ISTRT
00950 C
00960      1 IERR=1
00970        DO 250 I=1,100
00980    250 TILMRT(I)=TITL(I)
00990        TBMRT(1) = TBNO(1)
01000        TBMRT(2) = TBNO(2)
01010        DO 255 J=1,50
01020    255 ARAMRT(J) = AREA(J)
01030 C
01040 C      BRASS ESTIMATE OF MORTALITY
01050 C
01060        IF (ISTRT.EQ.1.AND.IEXIT.EQ.4) PRINT 60
01070        CALL BRASS(NW,NCEB,NCS,TILMRT,ARAMRT,TBMRT,NREG,LLVEL,IERR,LOAGE,
01080      1 IFIT, QSELEC,NQO,IPCH,SEXRAT)
01090 C
01100 C WHEN BRASS IS USED, CONSTANT MORTALITY IS ASSUMED
01110 C
01120        DO 260 I=1,15
01130        NNEG(I)=NREG
01140    260 LEVEL(I)=LLVEL
01150 C
01160 C      BRANCH ON ERROR CONDITION
01170        GO TO (300,300,999,999,999,999,999,999,999),IERR
01180 C      PROCEED ONLY IF IEXIT > 1
01190    300 IF (IEXIT-1) 700,700,310
01200    310 CONTINUE
01210        CALL LIFET(NNEG,LEVEL,TILMRT,ARAMRT,TBMRT,LIFTBF,LIFTBM,IPRIN2,
01220      1 ITP2,1,LLXF,LLXM,LLXF0,LLXM0)
01230        IF (NYEAR.LT.2) GO TO 390
01240        DO 350 I=2,NYEAR
01250        DO 330 J=1,18
01260        LIFTBF(J,I)=LIFTBF(J,1)
01270        LIFTBM(J,I)=LIFTBM(J,1)
01280    330 CONTINUE
```

Listing C.4. MAIN *(continued)*

```
01290        LLXF(I)=LLXF(1)
01300        LLXM(I)=LLXM(1)
01310        LLXFO(I)=LLXFO(1)
01320        LLXMO(I)=LLXMO(1)
01330    350 CONTINUE
01340  C
01350        GO TO 390
01360      2 CONTINUE
01370        READ(8,10420,END=992) ARAMRT,TBMRT,(TILMRT(K),K=1,60),
01380      1 (TILMRT(KK),KK=61,100),((NNEG(K),LEVEL(K)),K=1,15)
01390        PRINT 60
01400        PRINT 10420, ARAMRT,TBMRT,(TILMRT(K),K=1,60),
01410      1 (TILMRT(KK),KK=61,100),((NNEG(K),LEVEL(K)),K=1,15)
01420        DO 380 I=1,NYEAR
01430        NREG=NNEG(I)
01440        IF (NREG.LT.1.OR.NREG.GT.4) GO TO 994
01450    380 CONTINUE
01460  C
01470  C      CREATE 5-YEAR LIFE TABLES MALE AND FEMALE
01480  C
01490    400 CONTINUE
01500        CALL LIFET(NNEG,LEVEL,TILMRT,ARAMRT,TBMRT,LIFTBF,LIFTBM,IPRIN2,
01510      1 ITP2,NYEAR,LLXF,LLXM,LLXFO,LLXMO)
01520  C
01530  C
01540    390 CONTINUE
01550        IF (IEXIT-2) 700,700,500
01560      3 CONTINUE
01570        PRINT 60
01580        DO 410 I=1,NYEAR
01590        READ (8,10430,END=992) ARAMRT,TBMRT,TILMRT,(LIFTBF(J,I),J=1,18)
01600      1 (LIFTBM(K,I),K=1,18),LLXF(I),LLXM(I),LLXFO(I),LLXMO(I)
01610    410 CONTINUE
01620  C
01630  C      CALCULATE SURVIVAL RATIOS
01640  C
01650    500 CALL SURVIV(LIFTBF,LIFTBM,SR,IPRIN3,ITP3,TILMRT,ARAMRT,TBMRT,
01660      1 SEXRAT,NYEAR,LLXF,LLXM,LLXFO,LLXMO,IYEAR)
01670  C
01680        IF (IEXIT-3) 700,700,600
01690      4 CONTINUE
01700  C
01710  C
01720  C      READ SURVIVAL RATIOS
01730  C
01740  C
01750        READ (8,10440,END=992) ARAMRT,TBMRT,TILMRT
01760        PRINT 60
01770        PRINT 10440, ARAMRT,TBMRT,TILMRT
01780        DO 510 J=1,52
01790        READ(8,10450,END=992) (SR(I,J),I=1,16)
01800    510 CONTINUE
01810        PRINT 10455, SR
01820    600 CONTINUE
01830  C      OWN-CHILDREN FERTILITY ESTIMATION
01840  C
01850      5 CONTINUE
01860    550 CALL OWN (TAB,SR,UPPER,IUPC,ITP4,IPRIN4,IYEAR,TITL,TBNO,AREA,ST
01870      1 ENUM,ENUMW,NOWN,SUMARY)
01880        MRTFLG=1
01890    700 CONTINUE
01900        GO TO 100
01910    980 PRINT 9980
01920        GO TO 999
```

Listing C.4. MAIN *(continued)*

```
01930    990 PRINT 9990
01940        GO TO 999
01950    991 PRINT 9991
01960        GO TO 999
01970    992 PRINT 9992
01980        GO TO 999
01990    994 PRINT 9994,TBMRT,ARMRT,TILMRT,NREG,LEVEL(I)
02000        GO TO 999
02010    995 PRINT 9995
02020        GO TO 999
02030    996 PRINT 9996
02040        GO TO 999
02050    997 PRINT 9997
02060        GO TO 999
02070    998 PRINT 9998
02080     10 FORMAT (13I5,5X,F5.0)
02090     15 FORMAT('1FERTILITY ESTIMATION USING OWN-CHILDREN METHOD'/
02100        1' EAST-WEST POPULATION INSTITUTE, EAST-WEST CENTER'/
02110        2' VERSION 3.4 (JANUARY 1978)'///
02120        3    '   ISTRT  IEXIT QSELEC    NREG  LOAGE    IPCH   ITP2 IPRIN2
02130        4 ITP3 IPRIN3    ITP4    LP  NYEAR SEXRAT'/13I7,F7.2)
02140     20 FORMAT(20A4)
02150     40 FORMAT(1X,20A4)
02160     50 FORMAT (2I4,10(I3,1X,I2)/4(5X,15F5.0/),5X,6F5.0/5X,15F5.0/
02170        1     2(7F7.0/),5A4)
02180     60 FORMAT(1H1)
02190     70 FORMAT(///' CENSUS YEAR:',I5,'    MONTH:',I3//
02200        1' UNDER ENUMERATION FACTORS FOR CHILDREN'/6X,15F7.3//
02210        2' UNDER ENUMERATION FACTORS FOR WOMEN'/3(6X,15F7.3/),6X, 6F7.3//
02220        5' PROPORTION MARRIED'/6X,7F7.4//
02230        6' STANDARD POPULATION'/6X,7F7.0////
02240        9' STANDARDS ARE:'//6X,5A4,5X,'AS STANDARD POPULATION'/1H1)
02250     80 FORMAT(20A4)
02260     85 FORMAT(40X,20A4)
02270   9980 FORMAT(/' ERR009   ISTRT OR IEXIT INVALID ON PARAMETER CARD ' )
02280   9991 FORMAT(/' ERR002   STARTING POINT > EXIT POINT--ABEND')
02290   9990 FORMAT(/' ERR001   EOF ON PARAMETER INPUT STREAM--ABEND' )
02300   9992 FORMAT(/' ERR003   ENDFILE ON UNIT 8' )
02310   9994 FORMAT (/1X,2A1,1X,50A1/1X,100A1/' ERR005   ERROR ON REGION.   CODE
02320        1= ',I4,'   LEVEL = ',F6.2 )
02330   9995 FORMAT(/' ERR006   LOWEST AGE OF WOMEN FOR BRASS ESTIMATE OF MORTAL
02340        1ITY IS < 15 OR > 30 ' )
02350   9996 FORMAT(/' ERR007   ERROR ON PARAMETER CARD - RESERVED INPUT UNIT SE
02360        1LECTED FOR OUTPUT--ABEND' )
02370   9997 FORMAT(/' ERR008   ENDFILE ON UNIT 4 --   TABLE READING INCOMPLETE -
02380        1- ABEND ' )
02390   9998 FORMAT(' UPPER AGE OF WOMEN < 54 - ABEND')
02400  10420 FORMAT(1X,50A1,1X,2A1/12X,60A1/12X,40A1/10(I2,F6.2)/5(I2,F6.2))
02410  10430 FORMAT(1X,50A1,1X,2A1/12X,60A1/12X,40A1/(12X,6F10.0))
02420  10440  FORMAT(1X,50A1,1X,2A1 / 12X,60A1 / 12X,40A1,1X,A4,F6.2  )
02430  10450 FORMAT(12X,8F7.0/12X,8F7.0)
02440  10455 FORMAT (12X,8F7.4)
02450  10460 FORMAT(////)
02460    999 CONTINUE
02470        IF (ITP2.NE.0) ENDFILE ITP2
02480        IF (ITP3.NE.0) ENDFILE ITP3
02490        IF (ITP4.NE.6) ENDFILE ITP4
02500  C     END FILE 19
02510        PRINT 60
02520        STOP
02530        END
```

Input card deck set-up. The input cards are of three types: the parameter control card, the control cards for OWN, and the cards for FORTRAN unit number 8. The first input card for the OWCH3 program is the *parameter control card.* It provides parameters for program control, parameters used by the BRASS subroutine, and input–output device assignments (Table C.2).

Table C.2. Format of the parameter control card for OWCH3

Columns	Name	Contents	Format	Default
1–5	ISTRT	Entry point into the program package. It identifies which of the four steps will be processed first. 1=BRASS 2=LIFET 3=SURVIV 4=OWN	I5	1
6–10	IEXIT	Exit point of the package. It identifies the last step to be processed. 1=BRASS 2=LIFET 3=SURVIV 4=OWN IEXIT cannot be smaller than ISTRT.	I5	4
11–15	QSELEC	Parameter used in BRASS. It identifies which $_xq_0$ is to be used in estimating mortality and in selecting the closest regional model life table. $1=_2q_0$ $2=_3q_0$ $3=_5q_0$ 4=average $(_2q_0 + _3q_0)$ (default) 5=average $(_2q_0 + _5q_0)$	I5	4
16–20	NREG	Parameter used in BRASS. It is the region code for regional model life table to be selected by BRASS technique. 1=West (default) 2=North 3=East 4=South	I5	1
21–25	LOAGE	Paremeter used in BRASS. It is the lowest age of women in the first five-year age group. $15 \leqslant$ LOAGE $\leqslant 31$. In most cases the default value of 15 works well, but when the average age at first birth is unusually late, set LOAGE to the larger value.	I5	15
26–30	IPCH	Parameter passed to BRASS for optional punching of calculated q values, region, and selected level of regional model life table, plus identifying information. Output is in fixed format.	I5	0

Table C.2. *(continued)*

Columns	Name	Contents	Format	Default
31–35	ITP2	Parameter passed to LIFET. It is the FORTRAN unit number for optional output of female and male five-year regional model Life table L_x and labeling information. It cannot be 4, 5, or 8 (reserved for input). 0=no output. Output is in fixed format with a minimum record length of 80 bytes.	I5	0
36–40	IPRIN2	Parameter passed to LIFET for optional printing of female and male five-year regional model life tables and labeling information. 0=no output (default). 1=complete printout (1 page).	I5	0
41–45	ITP3	Parameter passed to SURVIV. It is similar to ITP2 and is FORTRAN unit number for optional output of survival ratios for children and women. It cannot be 4, 5, or 8 (reserved for input). 0=no output. Output is in fixed format with minimum record length of 80 bytes.	I5	0
46–50	IPRIN3	Parameter passed to SURVIV for optional printing of survival ratios, including labeling information. 0=no printout. 1=complete printout (1 page).	I5	0
51–55	ITP4	Parameter passed to OWN. It is similar to ITP2 and is FORTRAN unit number for optional output of complete own-children analysis. Output is as it would go to the line printer, complete with all labeling and identification. Minimum record length is 133 bytes. If no unit number is specified or if 0 is specified, the output is sent to the line printer. All other numbers are valid except 4, 5, and 6.	I5	0
56–60	LP1	Parameter used when the run includes calls to OWN. It indicates the number of times the program will loop through calls to OWN using the same set of survival ratios. The default will use a new set of survival ratios with each own-children table.	I5	1

Table C.2. *(continued)*

Columns	Name	Contents	Format	Default
61–65	NYEAR	Parameter passed to LIFET and SUR-VIV. It is the maximum number of years prior to the census for which birth rates are to be computed. If OWN is also called, NYEAR will be equal to the upper age of children plus 1. 1 ≤ NYEAR ≤ 15.	I5	15
71–75	SEXRAT	Parameter passed to BRASS and SURVIV. It is the sex ratio to be used in selecting the nearest regional model life table and in calculating survival ratios for children.	F5.0	1.05

A set of *control cards for OWN* is required following the parameter control card if IEXIT in the parameter control card is equal to 4. The format and content of the cards are shown in Table C.3.

Table C.3. Format of the control cards for OWN subroutine of OWCH3

Card number	Columns	Content
OWN1	1–4	IYEAR: year of the census
	5–8	MONTH: month of the census
		Range of calendar years for running averages of age-specific birth rates. Any number of ranges may be specified, up to the maximum of ten ranges. If no grouping is specified, default of five-year groupings will be computed.
	10–14	First range: e.g., 62–66
	16–20	Second range
	•	•
	•	•
	•	•
	64–68	Tenth range
OWN2	6–10	Enumeration correction factor for age 0, both sexes. Specify decimal point. (Correction factor × census count = true population.)
	11–15	Enumeration correction factor for age 1, both sexes. Specify decimal point.
	•	•
	•	•
	•	•

Table C.3. *(continued)*

Card number	Columns	Contents
	76–80	Enumeration correction factor for age 14, both sexes. Specify decimal point.
OWN3	6–10	Enumeration correction factor for age 15, female. Specify decimal point.
	11–15	Enumeration correction factor for age 16, female. Specify decimal point.
	•	•
	•	•
	•	•
	76–80	Enumeration correction factor for age 29, female. Specify decimal point.
OWN4	Same as card OWN3	for ages 30–44
OWN5	Same as card OWN3	for ages 45–59
OWN6	Same as card OWN3	for ages 60–65
OWN7	6–10	Non-own children factor for children of age 0. Specify decimal point. If the number of non-own children is included in the own-children tabulation, the non-own factors may be computed in the INPUT subroutine and replace the values on this card.
	11–15	Non-own children factor for children of age 1. Specify decimal point.
	•	•
	•	•
	•	•
	76–80	Non-own children factor for children age 14. Specify decimal point.
OWN8	1–7	Proportion of currently married women aged 15–19 at the time of the census. Specify decimal point.
	8–14	Proportion of currently married women aged 20–24 at the time of the census. Specify decimal point.
	•	•
	•	•
	•	•
	43–49	Proportion of currently married women aged 45–49 at the time of the census. Specify decimal point.
OWN9	1–7	Number of women aged 15–19 in a user-selected standard population
	8–14	Number of women aged 20–24 in a user-selected standard population
	•	•
	•	•
	•	•

Table C.3. *(continued)*

Card number	Columns	Contents
	43–49	Number of women aged 45–49 in a user-selected standard population
OWN10	1–20	Description of standard population used in card OWN9
OWN11–OWN15	1–80	Documentation information and comments. All five cards must be included even if some of them are blank.

Notes: 1. When there is no independent information on the adjustment factors on cards OWN2 through OWN7, the value 1.0 may be used.
2. Parameter control card through card OWN15 may be repeated as many times as the user desires.

FOR TRAN *unit number 8* is used to enter mortality data when ISTRT on the parameter control card is not equal to 1. The content and format of the data depend on the value of ISTRT on the parameter control card. When ISTRT = 3, the user must supply q_x columns, L_0 values, and L(last) values from the female and male life tables for each year, starting with the census year, back to the fifteenth year before the census. The content and format of the input cards are shown in Table C.4.

Table C.4. Format of the cards for FORTRAN unit number 8 in OWCH3

Card number	Columns	Content
1	2–51	Alpha–numeric area description
	76–77	Alpha–numeric table number
	78–80	Card sequence number (1)
2	2–11	First 10 characters of the alpha–numeric area description
	13–72	First 60 characters of the alpha–numeric description of input data
	76–77	Same as in card 1
	78–80	Card sequence number (2)
3	2–11	Same as in card 2
	13–52	Last 40 characters of the alpha–numeric description of input data
	76–77	Same as in card 1
	78–80	Card sequence number (3)

Table C.4. *(continued)*

Card number	Columns	Content
4	2–11	Same as in card 2
	13–22	$_1q_0$ for females for census year
	23–32	$_4q_1$ for females for census year
	33–42	$_5q_5$ for females for census year
	43–52	$_5q_{10}$ for females for census year
	53–62	$_5q_{15}$ for females for census year
	63–72	$_5q_{20}$ for females for census year
	76–77	Same as in card 1
	78–80	Card sequence number (4)
5		Same as card 4 for $_5q_{25}$ to $_5q_{50}$
6		Same as card 4 for $_5q_{55}$ to $_\infty q_{80}$
7,8,9		Same as cards 4–6 for males for census year
10		Same as card 4 for $L_{80}(f)$, $L_{80}(m)$, $_1L_0(f)$, $_1L_0(m)$
11–20		Same as cards 1–10 for year immediately preceding the census
•		
•		
•		
141–150		Same as cards 1–10 for fourteenth year preceding the census

Note: The q_x values are multiplied by the radix of the life table (usually 100,000) and entered without decimal points. The last age group for q_x may be smaller than 80+, provided that it is consistent with L_x on cards 10, 20, etc.

Input–Output devices. The OWCH3 program requires the following input–output devices: card reader (FORTRAN unit 5), printer (FORTRAN unit 6), FORTRAN unit 8 if $2 \leqslant$ ISTRT $\leqslant 4$, and FORTRAN units ITP2, ITP3, ITP4 if they are not defined to be 0 on the parameter control card. FORTRAN units ITP2, ITP3, and ITP4 may take the same value. FORTRAN unit 4 is reserved for the own-children tables, which are read by the subroutine INPUT. The card reader is reserved for parameter cards, and the unit 8 is reserved for mortality data. Note the ITP2, ITP3, and ITP4 cannot assume value 4, 5, or 8.

SURVIV. SURVIV is a FORTRAN program (Listing C.5) that computes survival ratios for children from birth to age i, and for women from age $a - i$ to age a, for $15 \leqslant a \leqslant 65$ and $0 \leqslant i \leqslant 14$. Input to the subroutine consists of male and female abridged life table $_nq_x$ values for each year for which fertility is to be estimated, sex ratio at birth, and other bookkeeping information. The program first interpolates abridged life tables into single-year life tables, following the procedure described in Appendix A, by calling subroutine INTER (not listed here). Then male and female life tables are combined using the sex ratio at birth. The combined single-year life tables are used to compute survival ratios of children, and the female single-year life tables are used to compute survival ratios of women. As mentioned earlier, reverse-survival ratios are obtained later by inverting the survival ratios.

Listing C.5. SURVIV

```
      SUBROUTINE  SURVIV(ALFTBF,ALFTBM,SR,IPRIN3,ITP3,TITL,ARA,        00000010
     1 TBNO,SEXRAT,NYEAR,LLXF,LLXM,LLXFO,LLXMO,IYEAR)                  00000020
      DIMENSION  FEMAL(100,15),SR(16,52),TITL(100),TBNO(2),AREA(10),   00000030
     1 ARA(50),EL(100),EOF(15),EOM(15),NNY(15)                        00000040
      INTEGER*4 UPPER                                                  00000050
      REAL*4 ALFTBF(18,15),ALFTBM(18,15),MALE(100,15),KO              00000060
      REAL*4 LLXF(15),LLXM(15),LLXFO(15),LLXMO(15)                     00000070
      SEXRP1=SEXRAT+1.0                                                00000080
      DO 10 I=1,10                                                     00000090
   10 AREA(I)=ARA(I)                                                   00000100
      DO 100 J=1,NYEAR                                                 00000110
C                                                                     00000120
C     COMPUTE 1(X) - FEMALE                                           00000130
C                                                                     00000140
      I=18                                                            00000150
   20 BASE=ALFTBF(I,J)                                                00000160
      IF (BASE.GT.0.0) GO TO 30                                       00000170
      I=I-1                                                           00000180
      GO TO 20                                                        00000190
   30 CONTINUE                                                        00000200
      DO 35 K=1,18                                                    00000210
      ALFTBF(K,J)=ALFTBF(K,J)/BASE                                    00000220
      ALFTBM(K,J)=ALFTBM(K,J)/BASE                                    00000230
   35 CONTINUE                                                        00000240
      EL(1)=100000.0                                                  00000250
      MAX=I                                                           00000260
      MAX1=MAX-1                                                      00000270
      MMAX=(MAX-2)*5                                                  00000280
      MMAX1=MMAX+1                                                    00000290
      Q0=ALFTBF(1,J)                                                  00000300
      EL(2)=EL(1)*(1.0-ALFTBF(1,J))                                   00000310
      EL(6)=EL(2)*(1.0-ALFTBF(2,J))                                   00000320
      DO 40 I=3,MAX                                                   00000330
      II=I*5-4                                                        00000340
   40 EL(II)=EL(II-5)*(1.0-ALFTBF(I,J))                               00000350
C                                                                     00000360
C     INTERPOLATE 1(X) - FEMALE                                       00000370
C                                                                     00000380
      CALL INTER(EL,Q0,MAX,1)                                         00000390
C                                                                     00000400
C     COMPUTE  L(X) - FEMALE                                          00000410
C                                                                     00000420
      KO=0.35                                                         00000430
      IF (Q0.LT.0.1)  KO=0.05+3.0*Q0                                  00000440
      FEMAL(1,J)=KO*EL(1)+ (1.0-KO)*EL(2)                             00000450
      DO 50  I=2,MMAX                                                 00000460
```

Listing C.5. SURVIV *(continued)*

```
      FEMAL(I,J)=0.5*EL(I)+0.5*EL(I+1)                        00000470
   50 CONTINUE                                                00000480
      FEMAL(MMAX1,J)=LLXF(J)                                  00000490
      IF (LLXF0(J).GT.0.0) FEMAL(1,J)=LLXF0(J)                00000500
C                                                             00000510
C     COMPUTE l(X) - MALE                                     00000520
C                                                             00000530
      Q0=ALFTBM(1,J)                                          00000540
      EL(2)=EL(1)*(1.0-ALFTBM(1,J))                           00000550
      EL(6)=EL(2)*(1.0-ALFTBM(2,J))                           00000560
      DO 60 I=3,MAX1                                          00000570
      II=I*5-4                                                00000580
   60 EL(II)=EL(II-5)*(1.0-ALFTBM(I,J))                       00000590
C                                                             00000600
C     INTERPOLATE l(X) - MALE                                 00000610
C                                                             00000620
      CALL INTER(EL,Q0,MAX,2)                                 00000630
C                                                             00000640
C     COMPUTE  L(X) - MALE                                    00000650
C                                                             00000660
      K0=0.33                                                 00000670
      IF (Q0.LT.0.1)  K0=0.0425+2.875*Q0                      00000680
      MALE (1,J)=K0*EL(1) + (1.0-K0)*EL(2)                    00000690
      DO 70 I=2,MMAX                                          00000700
      MALE(I,J)=0.5*EL(I) +0.5*EL(I+1)                        00000710
   70 CONTINUE                                                00000720
      MALE(MMAX1,J)=LLXM(J)                                   00000730
      IF (LLXM0(J).GT.0.0) MALE(1,J)=LLXM0(J)                 00000740
C                                                             00000750
C     COMPUTE LIFE EXPECTANCIES                               00000760
C                                                             00000770
  100 CONTINUE                                                00000780
      DO 75 J=1,NYEAR                                         00000790
      NNY(J)=IYEAR-J+1                                        00000800
      EOF(J)=0.0                                              00000810
      EOM(J)=0.0                                              00000820
      DO 74 I=1,MMAX1                                         00000830
      EOF(J)=EOF(J)+FEMAL(I,J)                                00000840
      EOM(J)=EOM(J)+MALE(I,J)                                 00000850
   74 CONTINUE                                                00000860
      EOF(J)=EOF(J)/100000.0                                  00000870
      EOM(J)=EOM(J)/100000.0                                  00000880
   75 CONTINUE                                                00000890
      WRITE (6,501) (NNY(J),J=1,NYEAR)                        00000900
      DO 76 I=1,MMAX1                                         00000910
      IAG=I-1                                                 00000920
      ID=(IAG/5)*5-IAG                                        00000930
      IF (ID.EQ.0) WRITE(6,901)                               00000940
   76 WRITE(6,601) IAG,(FEMAL(I,J),J=1,NYEAR)                 00000950
      WRITE(6,701) (EOF(J),J=1,NYEAR)                         00000960
      WRITE(6,801) (NNY(J),J=1,NYEAR)                         00000970
      DO 77 I=1,MMAX1                                         00000980
      IAG=I-1                                                 00000990
      ID=(IAG/5)*5-IAG                                        00001000
      IF (ID.EQ.0) WRITE(6,901)                               00001010
   77 WRITE(6,601) IAG,(MALE(I,J),J=1,NYEAR)                  00001020
      WRITE(6,701) (EOM(J),J=1,NYEAR)                         00001030
C                                                             00001040
C     COMPUTE SURVIVAL RATIOS                                 00001050
C                                                             00001060
      MAX=51+NYEAR                                            00001070
      DO 90 I=1,16                                            00001080
      IF  (I.LE.NYEAR)                                        00001090
```

Listing C.5. SURVIV *(continued)*

```
      1  SR(I,1)=((FEMAL(1,I)+SEXRAT*MALE(1,I))/SEXRP1)/1.0E05      00001100
         DO 80 J=2,52                                              00001110
         SR(I,J)=1.0                                               00001120
     80 CONTINUE                                                   00001130
     90 CONTINUE                                                   00001140
         DO 130 I=1,NYEAR                                          00001150
         IF(I.EQ.1) GO TO 115                                      00001160
         DO 110 J=2,I                                              00001170
         SR(I,1)=SR(I,1)*(FEMAL(I-J+2,J-1)+SEXRAT*MALE(I-J+2,J-1)) 00001180
      1 /(FEMAL(I-J+1,J-1)+SEXRAT*MALE(I-J+1,J-1))                 00001190
    110 CONTINUE                                                   00001200
    115 CONTINUE                                                   00001210
         DO 120 J=16,MAX                                           00001220
         K=J-14                                                    00001230
    120 SR(I+1,K)=SR(I,K)*FEMAL(J-I+1,I)/FEMAL(J-I,I)              00001240
    130 CONTINUE                                                   00001250
C       ZERO OUT ABOVE DIAGONAL ELEMENTS                          00001260
         DO 140 M=2,16                                             00001270
         DO 140 J=M,16                                             00001280
    140 SR(J,M) = 0.0                                              00001290
C                                                                  00001300
         IF (IPRIN3.EQ.0) GO TO 160                                00001310
         MAX=MAX-14                                                00001320
         NYEAR1=NYEAR+1                                            00001330
         PRINT 101, TBNO,ARA ,TITL,(II,II=1,15),(SR(I,1),I=1,NYEAR1) 00001340
         PRINT 1011                                                00001350
         DO 150 K=2,MAX                                            00001360
         IAGE = K + 13                                             00001370
    150 PRINT 201,IAGE,(SR(M,K),M=1,NYEAR1)                        00001380
    160 CONTINUE                                                   00001390
         IF (ITP3.EQ.0) RETURN                                     00001400
         WRITE (ITP3,301) ARA,TBNO,TBNO,AREA,(TITL(K),K=1,60),TBNO,AREA, 00001410
      1 (TITL(L),L=61,100),TBNO                                    00001420
         M = 2                                                     00001430
         DO 170 L=1,52                                             00001440
         M = M + 2                                                 00001450
         N = M + 1                                                 00001460
         WRITE(ITP3,401) AREA,(SR(K,L),K=1,8),TBNO,M,AREA,(SR(I,L),I=9,16),00001470
      2 TBNO,N                                                     00001480
    170 CONTINUE                                                   00001490
    101 FORMAT(1H1,1X,2A1,1X,50A1/1X,100A1//20X,                   00001500
      1 ' SURVIVAL RATIOS FOR CHIL',                              00001510
      1'DREN AGED 0-14 YEARS AND WOMEN AGED 15-65 YEARS BASED ON LIFE TAB00001520
      2LE' /7X,'0',15I8/ ' SURVIVAL RATIOS FOR CHILDREN FROM BIRTH TO AGE00001530
      3 I' / 16F8.5)                                              00001540
   1011 FORMAT(' SURVIVAL RATIOS FOR WOMEN FROM AGE A-I TO AGE A') 00001550
    201 FORMAT(I3,F5.1,15F8.5)                                     00001560
    301 FORMAT(1X,50A1,1X,2A1,21X,2A1,'   1' / 1X,10A1,1X,60A1,3X,2A1,'  2'00001570
      1 /1X,10A1,1X,40A1,23X,2A1,'   3')                          00001580
    401 FORMAT(1X,10A1,1X,8F7.5,7X,2A1,I3)                         00001590
    501 FORMAT(1H1,' FEMALE LIFE TABLE L(X) VALUES AND E0'///      00001600
      1 ' AGE',15I8/)                                             00001610
    601 FORMAT(I3,1X,15F8.0)                                       00001620
    701 FORMAT(/' E0 ',15F8.2)                                     00001630
    801 FORMAT(1H1,' MALE LIFE TABLE L(X) VALUES AND E0'///        00001640
      1 ' AGE',15I8/)                                             00001650
    901 FORMAT(/)                                                  00001660
   1002 FORMAT(10F10.0)                                            00001670
         RETURN                                                    00001680
         END                                                       00001690
         SUBROUTINE  INTER(EL,Q0,MAX,ISEX)                         00001700
         DIMENSION  EL(100),ALF(3,2),D(3,2)                        00001710
         DATA ALF/.489, .260, .112, .484, .258, .110/             00001720
         DATA D/.656, .601, .370, 1.353, 1.089, .571/             00001730
```

Listing C.5. SURVIV *(continued)*

```
C                                                                    00001740
      DO 10 I=3,5                                                    00001750
      K=I-2                                                          00001760
      AI=ALF(K,ISEX)                                                 00001770
      IF  (Q0.LT.0.1)  AI=AI+D(K,ISEX)*(0.1-Q0)                      00001780
      EL(I)=AI*EL(2)+(1.0-AI)*EL(6)                                  00001790
   10 CONTINUE                                                       00001800
      EL(7)=-0.5454545*EL(5)+1.44*EL(6)+0.12*EL(11)-0.01454545*EL(16) 00001810
      EL(8)=-0.7272727*EL(5)+1.44*EL(6)+0.32*EL(11)-0.0327272727*EL(16) 00001820
      EL(9)=-0.6363636*EL(5)+1.12*EL(6)+0.56*EL(11)-0.043636364*EL(16) 00001830
      EL(10)=-0.3636364*EL(5)+0.6*EL(6)+0.8*EL(11)-0.03636364*EL(16) 00001840
      MAX5=MAX-5                                                     00001850
      DO 20 I=1,MAX5                                                 00001860
      I1=(I+1)*5+2                                                   00001870
      K1=I1-6                                                        00001880
      K2=I1-1                                                        00001890
      K3=I1+4                                                        00001900
      K4=I1+9                                                        00001910
      EL(I1)=-0.048*EL(K1)+0.864*EL(K2)+0.216*EL(K3)-0.032*EL(K4)    00001920
      EL(I1+1)=-0.064*EL(K1)+0.672*EL(K2)+0.448*EL(K3)-0.056*EL(K4)  00001930
      EL(I1+2)=-0.056*EL(K1)+0.448*EL(K2)+0.672*EL(K3)-0.064*EL(K4)  00001940
      EL(I1+3)=-0.032*EL(K1)+0.216*EL(K2)+0.864*EL(K3)-0.048*EL(K4)  00001950
   20 CONTINUE                                                       00001960
      I1=(MAX-3)*5+2                                                 00001970
      K1=I1-11                                                       00001980
      K2=I1-6                                                        00001990
      K3=I1-1                                                        00002000
      K4=I1+4                                                        00002010
      EL(I1)=0.032*EL(K1)-0.176*EL(K2)+1.056*EL(K3)+0.088*EL(K4)     00002020
      EL(I1+1)=0.056*EL(K1)-0.288*EL(K2)+1.008*EL(K3)+0.224*EL(K4)   00002030
      EL(I1+2)=0.064*EL(K1)-0.312*EL(K2)+0.832*EL(K3)+0.416*EL(K4)   00002040
      EL(I1+3)=0.048*EL(K1)-0.224*EL(K2)+0.504*EL(K3)+0.672*EL(K4)   00002050
      RETURN                                                         00002060
      END                                                            00002070
```

The SURVIV subroutine is called by the statement:

CALL SURVIV(LIFTBF,LIFTBM,SR,IPRIN3,ITP3,TITLE, AREA,TBNO,SEXRAT,NYEAR).

The parameters of the subroutine are:

LIFTBF(18,15)   REAL
Given array of $_nq_x$'s from female abridged life tables for 0–14 years prior to the census, where LIFTBF($*,j+1$) contains 18 $_nq_x$ values ($x=0,1,5,...80$) for year j prior to the census. $0 \leqslant j \leqslant 14$.

LIFTBM(18,15)   REAL
Given array of $_nq_x$'s from male abridged life tables for 0–14 years prior to the census, where LIFTBM($*,j+1$) contains 18 $_nq_x$ values ($x=0,1,5,...80$) for year j prior to the census. $0 \leqslant j \leqslant 14$.

SR(16,52)	REAL
	Resultant survival ratios for children and women.

SR(i+1,1):   Survival ratios for children from birth to age i; $0 \leqslant i \leqslant 15$.

SR(i+1,a–13):   Survival ratios for women from age a–i to age i; $15 \leqslant a \leqslant 65$, $0 \leqslant i \leqslant 15$.

IPRIN3   INTEGER
Given parameter for complete printing of survival ratios table with headings. 0 indicates no printout of survival ratios, and 1 indicates a full-page printout of survival ratios.

ITP3   INTEGER
Given FORTRAN unit number for optional output of survival ratios and labeling information.

TITLE(100)   REAL
Given title or other identification. Used in format 100A1.

AREA(50)   REAL
Given area description. First ten characters may be an area code. Used in format 50A1.

TBNO(2)   REAL
Given table number. Used in format 2A1.

SEXRAT   REAL
Given sex ratio at birth.

NYEAR   INTEGER
Given. (NYEAR–1) is the maximum number of years prior to the census that women and children will be reverse-survived.

When ITP3 is not zero, the computed survival ratios are saved on the FORTRAN unit ITP3 as punched card images using the following format:

Card no.	Content	Format
1–3	Title and information and card sequence number.	(77A1,I3)
4	Area code, survival ratios for children aged 0–7, table number, and card sequence number.	(1X,10A1,1X,8F7.6, 7X,2A1,I3)
5	Area code, survival ratios for children aged 8–14, table number, and card sequence number.	(1X,10A1,1X,7F7.6, 14X,2A1,I3)
6–107	Area code, survival ratios for women aged 15–65, table number, and card sequence number. There are two cards for each single year of age of women, starting with age 15. Thus cards 6 and 7 refer to women age 15, 8 and 9 to women age 16, etc.	

OWN. OWN is a FORTRAN program that computes single-year and five-year age-specific birth rates for each year back to the fifteenth year before the census. Input for this subroutine consists of the table of own children, the table of survival ratios for women and children, enumeration-adjustment factors for women and children, adjustment factors for unmatched children, and other bookkeeping information. Optional inputs are proportions of ever-married women for each five-year age group of women, for computing age-specific marital birth rates for one year immediately preceding the census, and number of women in each five-year age group in a standard population, for computing standardized general fertility rates. Outputs of this program are the following tables:

1. Live births by single years of age of mothers for each year preceding the census back to the fifteenth year before the census
2. Women by single years of age in the childbearing ages for each year preceding the census back to the fifteenth year before the census
3. Single-year age-specific birth rates, derived from the first two tables
4. Five-year age-specific birth rates, total fertility rates, general fertility rates, and age-standardized general fertility rates. These rates are presented for each calendar year preceding the census and for groups of calendar years as specified by the user. For the year preceding the census, five-year age-specific marital birth rates and the total marital fertility rate are computed as well.

The subroutine is called by the statement:

CALL OWN(TAB,SR,UPPER,IUPC,ITP4,IPRIN4,IYEAR,
TITLE,TBNO,AREA,STRD,ENUM,ENUMW,NOWN,SUMARY).

The parameters of the subroutine are:

TAB(16,51)   REAL
Given women and own-children table.
TAB(1,a–14):   Total women of age a,
$15 \leqslant a \leqslant 65$.
TAB(2+i,a–14):   Own-children of age i to
women of age a, $0 \leqslant i \leqslant 14$.

SR(16,52)   REAL
Given survival ratios for women from age a–i to
age a, and for children from birth to age i.
SR(i+1,1):   Survival ratios for children.
SR(i+1,a–14):   Survival ratios for women
$15 \leqslant a \leqslant 65$, $0 \leqslant i \leqslant 15$.

UPPER   INTEGER
Given upper age of women in own-children
table.
UPPER$\leqslant$65.

IUPC   INTEGER
Given upper age of children in own-children
table.
IUPC$\leqslant$14.

ITP4   INTEGER
Given FORTRAN unit number for optional output of birth rates.

IPRIN4   INTEGER
Given parameter for complete printing of results. 0 indicates no printing and 1 indicates
complete printing.

IYEAR   INTEGER
Given year of the census.

TITLE(100)   REAL
Given title or other identification. Used in format 100A1.

TBNO(2)   REAL
Given table number. Used in format 2A1.

AREA(50)   REAL
Given area description. First ten characters may
be an area code. Used in format 50A1.

STRD(7,2)   REAL
Given proportions married and standard population by five-year age group of women for ages
15–49. Used in the calculation of the marital fertility rates and the standardized general fertility
rate.
STRD(*,1):   Proportions married at time of
            the census.
STRD(*,2):   Number of women in a user-
            selected standard population.

ENUM(15)   REAL
Given enumeration adjustment factors by age of
child. Enumerated counts are multiplied by the
adjustment factors.
ENUM(i+1):   Enumeration adjustment fac-
              tor for children of age i,
              $0 \leqslant i \leqslant 14$.

ENUMW(51)   REAL
Given enumeration adjustment factors by age of
women. Enumerated counts are multiplied by
the adjustment factors.
ENUMW(a–14): Enumeration adjustment fac-
              tor for women of age a,
              $15 \leqslant a \leqslant 65$.

NOWN(15)   REAL
Given non-own factors by age of child, used to
inflate the tabulated number of own children to
adjust for children not living with their mothers
at the time of the census.
NOWN(i+1):   Non-own factor for children
              age i, $0 \leqslant i \leqslant 14$.

SUMARY(2,10)   INTEGER
Used to compute summary fertility rates. The
summary rates for maximum of ten time periods
will be computed for years SUMARY(1,*) to
SUMARY(2,*).

Listing C.6. OWN

```
      SUBROUTINE OWN(TAB,SR,UPPER,IUPC,ITP4,IPRIN4,IYEAR,TITLE,TBNO,      00000010
     1 AREA,STRD,ENUM,ENUMW,NOWN,SUMARY)                                  00000020
      DIMENSION TAB(16,51),CHLD(16,52),WMN(16,52),SR(16,52),STRD(7,2),    00000030
     1ENUM(15),ENUMW(51),BR(5,8),TITLE(100),TBNO(2),AREA(50),NYEAR(16),   00000040
     2 SUMRYB(8,10),SUMRYW(7,10),IDT(6),ADJ(15,51)                        00000050
      REAL*4 NOWN(15)                                                     00000060
      INTEGER*4 UW,UC,UPPER,IUPC,UCM1,UWM1,SUMARY(2,10)                   00000070
      DIMENSION TCHLD(51),TWMN(51),CWMN(16,52),TOTCH(16),TA(16)           00000080
C                                                                         00000090
C     SET BOUNDS FOR ARRAYS BASED ON MAX AGES                            00000100
C                                                                         00000110
      UW = UPPER-13                                                       00000120
      UC = IUPC+2                                                         00000130
      UCM1=IUPC+1                                                         00000140
      UWM1=UPPER-14                                                       00000150
      M2 = UWM1-1                                                         00000160
C                                                                         00000170
C                                                                         00000180
C     STANDARDS BY 5 YEAR AGE GROUP OF WOMEN                             00000190
C     1 - PROP MARRIED AT TIME OF CENSUS; 2 - NUMBER OF WOMEN IN A       00000200
C     STANDARD POPULATION.                                               00000210
C                                                                         00000220
C     INITIALIZE AND CALC                                               00000230
C                                                                         00000240
C                                                                         00000250
      WMN(1,UW)=0                                                         00000260
      CHLD(1,UW)=0                                                        00000270
      DO 10 I=1,UWM1                                                      00000280
      CHLD(1,I)=TAB(1,I)                                                  00000290
      CHLD(1,UW)=CHLD(1,UW)+CHLD(1,I)                                     00000300
      WMN(1,I)=TAB(1,I)* ENUMW(I)                                         00000310
   10 WMN(1,UW)=WMN(1,UW)+WMN(1,I)                                        00000320
      DO 11 I=2,UC                                                        00000330
      CHLD(I,UW)=0.0                                                      00000340
   11 WMN(I,UW) = 0.0                                                     00000350
C                                                                         00000360
      DO 25 K=1,16                                                        00000370
   25 NYEAR(K) = IYEAR-K + 1                                              00000380
C                                                                         00000390
C     BIRTHS AND REVERSE SURVIVED WOMEN                                  00000400
C                                                                         00000410
      DO 36 I=2,UC                                                        00000420
      K = I-1                                                             00000430
      TA(K)=0.0                                                           00000440
      TOTCH(K)=0.0                                                        00000450
      DO 30 J=1,UWM1                                                      00000460
      TOTCH(K)=TOTCH(K)+TAB(I,J)                                          00000470
      TA(K)=TA(K)+TAB(I,J)*ENUMW(J)                                       00000480
   30 CONTINUE                                                            00000490
      DO 35 J=1,UWM1                                                      00000500
      IF (TA(K).LE.0.0) GO TO 310                                         00000510
      ADJ(K,J)=ENUMW(J)*ENUM(K)*TOTCH(K)/TA(K)                           00000520
      GO TO 320                                                           00000530
  310 ADJ(K,J)=ENUM(K)                                                    00000540
  320 CONTINUE                                                            00000550
      L = J + 1                                                           00000560
      CHLD(I,J)=(TAB(I,J)/SR(K,1))*NOWN(K)*ADJ(K,J)                       00000570
      IF (SR(I,L).EQ.0) GO TO 31                                          00000580
      WMN(I,J)=TAB(1,J)/SR(I,L)*ENUMW(J)                                  00000590
      GO TO 32                                                            00000600
   31 WMN(I,J) = 0.0                                                      00000610
   32 WMN(I,UW)=WMN(I,UW)+WMN(I,J)                                        00000620
```

Listing C.6. OWN *(continued)*

```
   35 CHLD(I,UW)=CHLD(I,UW) + CHLD(I,J)                         00000630
   36 CONTINUE                                                  00000640
C                                                               00000650
C     PRINT BIRTH MATRIX AND REVERSE-SURVIVED WOMEN             00000660
C                                                               00000670
      WRITE (ITP4,1000) TBNO,AREA,TITLE,(K,K=1,IUPC)            00000680
      WRITE(ITP4,1010) (NYEAR(M),M=1,UCM1)                      00000690
      IAGE = 14                                                 00000700
      DO 40 K=1,UWM1                                            00000710
      IAGE = IAGE + 1                                           00000720
   40 WRITE(ITP4,1020) IAGE,WMN(1,K),(CHLD(I,K),I=2,UC)         00000730
      WRITE(ITP4,1030) WMN(1,UW),(CHLD(I,UW),I=2,UC)            00000740
      WRITE(ITP4,1040) (NOWN(L),L=1,UCM1)                       00000750
C                                                               00000760
      WRITE (ITP4,1100) TBNO,AREA,TITLE,(K,K=1,UCM1)            00000770
      WRITE(ITP4,1110) (NYEAR(M),M=1,UC)                        00000780
      IAGE = 14                                                 00000790
      DO 50 K=1,UWM1                                            00000800
      IAGE = IAGE + 1                                           00000810
   50 WRITE(ITP4,1520) IAGE,(WMN(I,K),I=1,UC)                   00000820
      WRITE(ITP4,1120) (WMN(I,UW),I=1,UC)                       00000830
C                                                               00000840
C     CENTRAL BIRTHS, WOMEN, AND FERTILITY                      00000850
C                                                               00000860
      DO 68 I=2,UC                                              00000870
      SUMM = 0                                                  00000880
      DO 65 J=1,M2                                              00000890
      K = J+I-1                                                 00000900
      IF (K.GT.UWM1) GO TO 58                                   00000910
      SUM=WMN(I,K)+WMN(I-1,K-1)                                 00000920
      TCHLD(J)=CHLD(I,K)+CHLD(I,K-1)                            00000930
      IF (SUM.EQ.0) GOTO 60                                     00000940
      TAB(I,J)=TCHLD(J)/SUM*1.0E03                              00000950
      GO TO 63                                                  00000960
   58 SUM=0.0                                                   00000970
   60 TAB(I,J)=0.0                                              00000980
   63 CONTINUE                                                  00000990
      CHLD(I,J)=TCHLD(J)*0.5                                    00001000
      CWMN(I,J)=SUM*0.5                                         00001010
   65 SUMM = SUMM + TAB(I,J)                                    00001020
      TAB(I,UWM1) = SUMM                                        00001030
   68 CONTINUE                                                  00001040
C                                                               00001050
C     PRINT CENTRAL BIRTH AND WOMEN MATRICES                    00001060
C                                                               00001070
      WRITE(ITP4,1500) TBNO,AREA,TITLE,(K,K=1,IUPC)             00001080
      WRITE(ITP4,1510) (NYEAR(M),M=1,UCM1)                      00001090
      IAGE=14                                                   00001100
      DO 2070 K=1,M2                                            00001110
      IAGE=IAGE+1                                               00001120
 2070 WRITE(ITP4,1520) IAGE,(CHLD(I,K),I=2,UC)                  00001130
      WRITE(ITP4,1600) TBNO,AREA,TITLE,(K,K=1,IUPC)             00001140
      WRITE(ITP4,1510) (NYEAR(M),M=1,UCM1)                      00001150
      IAGE=14                                                   00001160
      DO 2071 K=1, M2                                           00001170
      IAGE=IAGE+1                                               00001180
 2071 WRITE(ITP4,1520) IAGE,(CWMN(I,K),I=2,UC)                  00001190
C                                                               00001200
C     PRINT SINGLE YEAR ASFR                                    00001210
C                                                               00001220
      WRITE (ITP4,1200) TBNO,AREA,TITLE,(K,K=1,IUPC)            00001230
      WRITE(ITP4,1210) (NYEAR(M),M=1,UCM1)                      00001240
      IAGE = 14                                                 00001250
      DO 70 K=1,M2                                              00001260
```

Listing C.6. OWN *(continued)*

```
        IAGE = IAGE + 1                                              00001270
    70 WRITE(ITP4,1220) IAGE,(TAB(I,K),I=2,UC)                       00001280
       WRITE(ITP4,1230) (TAB(I,UWM1),I=2,UC)                         00001290
C                                                                    00001300
C       ZERO OUT ARRAY FOR STORAGE OF 5-YEAR RATES                   00001310
C                                                                    00001320
       LIM = 2*UCM1+2                                                00001330
       DO 80 I=1,9                                                   00001340
       DO 80 J=1,LIM                                                 00001350
    80 TAB(I,J)=0.0                                                  00001360
C                                                                    00001370
C       STORE BIRTHS BELOW WOMEN                                     00001380
C       ASFR BELOW WOMEN AND BIRTHS                                  00001390
C                                                                    00001400
       DO 150 II=2,UC                                                00001410
       I=II-1                                                        00001420
       M=I+UC                                                        00001430
       N=M+UC                                                        00001440
       TOTB=0.0                                                      00001450
       TOTW=0.0                                                      00001460
       DO 85 J=1,7                                                   00001470
       L = 5*(J-1)+ 1                                                00001480
       TAB(J,I)= CWMN(II,L)                                          00001490
       TAB(J,M)= CHLD(II,L)                                          00001500
       DO 82 K=1,4                                                   00001510
       TAB(J,I)=TAB(J,I)+CWMN(II,L+K)                                00001520
    82 TAB(J,M)=TAB(J,M)+CHLD(II,L+K)                                00001530
C                                                                    00001540
C       CHECK SO DON'T USE NON-EXIST. DATA                           00001550
C                                                                    00001560
       IF (UPPER-49.LT.I.AND.J.EQ.7) TAB(7,I)=0.0                    00001570
       IF (UPPER-49.LT.I.AND.J.EQ.7) TAB(7,M)=0.0                    00001580
    84 TOTB=TOTB+TAB(J,M)                                            00001590
    85 TOTW=TOTW+TAB(J,I)                                            00001600
       TAB(8,I)=TOTW                                                 00001610
       TAB(8,M)=TOTB                                                 00001620
C                                                                    00001630
C       CALCULATE 5-YEAR RATES                                       00001640
C                                                                    00001650
       TAB(8,N)=0.0                                                  00001660
       DO 95 J=1,7                                                   00001670
       IF (TAB(J,I).EQ.0.0) GO TO 92                                 00001680
       TAB(J,N)=TAB(J,M)/TAB(J,I)*1.0E03                             00001690
       GO TO 93                                                      00001700
    92 TAB(J,N)=0.0                                                  00001710
    93 CONTINUE                                                      00001720
       TAB(8,N)=TAB(8,N)+TAB(J,N)                                    00001730
    95 CONTINUE                                                      00001740
C                                                                    00001750
C       TFR                                                          00001760
C                                                                    00001770
       TAB(9,N)=(TAB(8,N)-TAB(7,N))*5.                               00001780
       TAB(8,N)=TAB(8,N)*5.0                                         00001790
C                                                                    00001800
C       GFR                                                          00001810
C                                                                    00001820
       IF (TAB(8,I).EQ.0.0) GO TO 103                                00001830
       TAB(10,N)=TAB(8,M)/TAB(8,I)*1.0E03                            00001840
       TAB(11,N)=(TAB(8,M)-TAB(7,M))/(TAB(8,I)-TAB(7,I))*1.0E03      00001850
       GO TO 104                                                     00001860
   103 TAB(10,N)=0.0                                                 00001870
       TAB(11,N)=0.0                                                 00001880
   104 CONTINUE                                                      00001890
C                                                                    00001900
```

Listing C.6. OWN *(continued)*

```
C      AGE STANDARDIZED GFR                                    00001910
C                                                              00001920
       XG = 0                                                  00001930
       XGSTR=0                                                 00001940
       TW = 0                                                  00001950
       DO 110 L=1,7                                            00001960
       XG=XG+TAB(L,N)*STRD(L,2)                                00001970
       TW=TW+STRD(L,2)                                         00001980
       IF (L.EQ.6) XGSTR=XG                                    00001990
   110 CONTINUE                                                00002000
       TAB(12,N)=XG/TW                                         00002010
       TAB(13,N)=XGSTR/(TW-STRD(7,2))                          00002020
   150 CONTINUE                                                00002030
C                                                              00002040
C      MARITAL FERTILITY                                       00002050
C                                                              00002060
       TAB(8,49)=0.0                                           00002070
       N=1+UC+UC                                               00002080
       DO 120 L=1,7                                            00002090
       TAB(L,49)=TAB(L, N)/STRD(L,1)                           00002100
   120 CONTINUE                                                00002110
C                                                              00002120
C      PRINT 5-YEAR BIRTHS AND WOMEN MATRICES                  00002130
C                                                              00002140
       WRITE (ITP4,1700) TBNO,AREA,TITLE,(K,K=1,IUPC)          00002150
       WRITE(ITP4,1710) (NYEAR(M),M=1,UCM1)                    00002160
       IUC1=UC+1                                               00002170
       IUC2=UC+UC-1                                            00002180
       IUC3=IUC2+2                                             00002190
       IUC4=IUC3+UC-2                                          00002200
       IUC5=IUC3+1                                             00002210
       IAG1=10                                                 00002220
       DO 210 I=1,7                                            00002230
       IAG1=IAG1+5                                             00002240
       IAG2=IAG1+4                                             00002250
   210 WRITE(ITP4,1720) IAG1,IAG2, (TAB(I,K),K=IUC1,IUC2)      00002260
       WRITE (ITP4,1800)                                       00002270
       IAG1=10                                                 00002280
       DO 220 I=1,7                                            00002290
       IAG1=IAG1+5                                             00002300
       IAG2=IAG1+4                                             00002310
   220 WRITE(ITP4,1720) IAG1,IAG2,(TAB(I,K),K=1,UCM1)          00002320
C                                                              00002330
C      PRINT OUT FIVE YEAR RATES                               00002340
C                                                              00002350
       WRITE(ITP4,1900) TBNO,AREA,TITLE,(K,K=1,IUPC)           00002360
       WRITE(ITP4,1910) (NYEAR(M),M=1,UCM1)                    00002370
       IAG1=10                                                 00002380
       DO 230 I=1,7                                            00002390
       IAG1=IAG1+5                                             00002400
       IAG2=IAG1+4                                             00002410
   230 WRITE(ITP4,1920) IAG1,IAG2, TAB(I,IUC3),TAB(I,49),      00002420
      1 (TAB(I,K),K=IUC5,IUC4)                                 00002430
       WRITE (ITP4,1930)  TAB(8,IUC3),        (TAB(8,K),K=IUC5,IUC4) 00002440
       WRITE (ITP4,1940) (TAB(9,K),K=IUC3,IUC4)                00002450
       WRITE (ITP4,1950) (TAB(10,K),K=IUC3,IUC4)               00002460
       WRITE (ITP4,1960) (TAB(11,K),K=IUC3,IUC4)               00002470
       WRITE (ITP4,1970) (TAB(12,K),K=IUC3,IUC4)               00002480
       WRITE (ITP4,1980) (TAB(13,K),K=IUC3,IUC4)               00002490
C                                                              00002500
C      SUMMARY FERTILITY RATES                                 00002510
C                                                              00002520
C      SUMMARY INDICES OK?                                     00002530
C                                                              00002540
```

Listing C.6. OWN *(continued)*

```
            MAXYR=IYEAR-1900                                              00002550
            MINYR=IYEAR-UCM1+1-1900                                       00002560
      160 CONTINUE                                                        00002570
            DO 161 I=1,10                                                 00002580
            IF (SUMARY(1,I).LT.MINYR) GO TO 162                           00002590
            IF (SUMARY(2,I).GT.MAXYR) GO TO 162                           00002600
            IF (SUMARY(1,I).GT.SUMARY(2,I)) GO TO 162                     00002610
      161 CONTINUE                                                        00002620
            I=11                                                          00002630
      162 NSUMRY=I-1                                                      00002640
            IF (NSUMRY.GE.1) GO TO 163                                    00002650
            SUMARY(1,1)=MINYR                                             00002660
            SUMARY(1,2)=MINYR+5                                           00002670
            SUMARY(1,3)=MINYR+10                                          00002680
            SUMARY(2,1)=MINYR+4                                           00002690
            SUMARY(2,2)=MINYR+9                                           00002700
            SUMARY(2,3)=MINYR+14                                          00002710
            GO TO 160                                                     00002720
    C                                                                     00002730
    C       SUMMARY BIRTHS AND WOMEN                                      00002740
    C                                                                     00002750
      163 CONTINUE                                                        00002760
            DO 166 J=1,NSUMRY                                             00002770
            SUMRYB(8,J)=0.0                                              00002780
            DO 165 I=1,7                                                  00002790
            SUMRYB(I,J)=0.0                                              00002800
            SUMRYW(I,J)=0.0                                              00002810
            I1=MAXYR-SUMARY(2,J)+1                                       00002820
            I2=MAXYR-SUMARY(1,J)+1                                       00002830
            DO 164  K=I1,I2                                               00002840
            SUMRYB(I,J)=SUMRYB(I,J)+TAB(I,IUC1+K-1)                      00002850
      164 SUMRYW(I,J)=SUMRYW(I,J)+TAB(I,K)                              00002860
            SUMRYB(I,J)=1000.0*SUMRYB(I,J)/SUMRYW(I,J)                   00002870
      165 SUMRYB(8,J)=SUMRYB(8,J)+SUMRYB(I,J)                           00002880
      166 SUMRYB(8,J)=SUMRYB(8,J)*5.0                                   00002890
            WRITE (ITP4,1400) TBNO,AREA,TITLE,((SUMARY(K,L),K=1,2),L=1,NSUMRY)00002900
            WRITE (ITP4,1990)                                            00002910
            KAGE = 15                                                    00002920
            DO 170 I=1,7                                                  00002930
            IAGE = KAGE +4                                                00002940
            WRITE(ITP4,1410) KAGE,IAGE,(SUMRYB(I,L),L=1,NSUMRY)          00002950
      170 KAGE=IAGE+1                                                     00002960
            WRITE(ITP4,1420) (SUMRYB(8,L),L=1,NSUMRY)                    00002970
    C                                                                     00002980
    C                                                                     00002990
    C                                                                     00003000
    C       PRINT OUT SUMMARY INFO IF SAVING ON TAPE                      00003010
    C                                                                     00003020
            TFROUT=TAB(8,IUC3)                                           00003030
            GFROUT=TAB(10,IUC3)                                          00003040
            IF (ITP4.NE.6) PRINT 5000,TBNO,AREA,TITLE,IYEAR,TFROUT,GFROUT 00003050
    C                                                                     00003060
    C                                                                     00003070
     1000 FORMAT(1H1,51X,'PERIOD-COHORT BIRTH MATRIX (BT)'/16X,           00003080
          1'EQUATION USED = CHILD / MORTALITY ADJUSTMENT FACTOR * NON-OWN FAC00003090
          XTOR * UNDER-ENUMERATION FACTOR'//1X,2A1,1X,50A1               00003100
          2/1X,100A1//41X,                                               00003110
          3 'NUMBER OF YEARS PRECEDING THE ','CENSUS'/28X,'<1 ',15I7)     00003120
     1010 FORMAT(' SURVEY',8X,'ALL'/2X,'AGE',9X,'WOMEN',6X,15I7)          00003130
     1020 FORMAT(2X,I2,6X,F9.1,6X,15F7.0)                                 00003140
     1030 FORMAT(1X,'TOTAL',4X,F9.0,6X,15F7.0)                           00003150
     1040 FORMAT(/1X,'NON-OWN FACTOR',10X,15F7.4)                        00003160
     1100 FORMAT(1H1,40X,'PERIOD-COHORT REVERSE SURVIVED WOMEN MATRIX (WT)' 00003170
          1/29X,'EQUATION USED: WOMEN / MORTALITY ADJUSTMENT FACTOR * ENUMERA00003180
```

Listing C.6. OWN *(continued)*

```
      XTION FACTOR'//1X,                                             00003190
     2 2A1,1X,50A1 / 1X,100A1 // 41X,'NUMBER OF YEARS PRECEDING THE ',  00003200
     3 'CENSUS' / 20X, '<1',15I7)                                   00003210
 1110 FORMAT (' SURVEY'/2X,'AGE',10X,16I7)                          00003220
 1120 FORMAT (1X,'TOTAL',9X,16F7.0)                                 00003230
 1200 FORMAT(1H1 / 35X,'ESTIMATED SINGLE-YEAR CENTRAL AGE-SPECIFIC FERTI00003240
     1LITY RATES(FC)' // 1X,2A1,1X,50A1 / 1X,100A1 // 41X,          00003250
     3 'NUMBER OF YEARS PRECEDING THE ','CENSUS' / 28X,'<1',14I7)   00003260
 1210 FORMAT(9X,'AGE OF'/ 10X,'WOMEN',9X,15I7)                      00003270
 1220 FORMAT(12X,I2,10X,15F7.1)                                     00003280
 1230 FORMAT(12X,'TFR',9X,15F7.1)                                   00003290
 1400 FORMAT(9(/),52X,'SUMMARY RATES'//1X,2A1,1X,50A1 / 1X,100A1 // 00003300
     1 3X,'WOMEN''S'/ 5X,'AGE',21X,10(I4,'-',I2))                   00003310
 1410 FORMAT ( I6,'-',I2,20X,10F7.1)                                00003320
 1420 FORMAT(/5X,'TFR   (15-49)',12X,10F7.1)                        00003330
 1500 FORMAT(1H1,51X,'CENTRAL SINGLE YEAR BIRTH MATRIX'///          00003340
     1 1X,2A1,1X,50A1/1X,100A1//47X,                               00003350
     2 'NUMBER OF YEARS PRECEDING THE',' CENSUS'/20X,'<1' ,14I7)    00003360
 1510 FORMAT(' WOMEN''S'/2X,'AGE',10X,15I7)                         00003370
 1520 FORMAT(2X,I2,11X,16F7.0)                                      00003380
 1600 FORMAT( 1H1,51X,'CENTRAL SINGLE YEAR WOMEN MATRIX'///         00003390
     1 1X,2A1,1X,50A1/1X,100A1//47X,                               00003400
     2 'NUMBER OF YEARS PRECEDING THE',' CENSUS'/20X,'<1' ,14I7)    00003410
 1700 FORMAT(1H1,51X,'CENTRAL 5-YEAR BIRTH MATRIX'///               00003420
     1 1X,2A1,1X,50A1/1X,100A1/45X,                                00003430
     2 'NUMBER OF YEARS PRECEDING THE',' CENSUS'/14X,'<1 ',14I8/)   00003440
 1710 FORMAT(' WOMEN''S'/3X,'AGE',4X,15I8/)                         00003450
 1720 FORMAT(I4,'-',I2,3X,15F8.0)                                   00003460
 1800 FORMAT(////57X,'CENTRAL 5-YEAR WOMEN MATRIX'//)               00003470
 1900 FORMAT(1H1,39X,'5-YEAR CENTRAL AGE-SPECIFIC FERTILITY RATES'///  00003480
     1 1X,2A1,1X,50A1/1X,100A1/45X,                                00003490
     2 'NUMBER OF YEARS PRECEDING THE',' CENSUS'/18X,'<1',8X,14I7/) 00003500
 1910 FORMAT(3X,'WOMEN''S'/5X,'AGE',6X,I8,' MARITAL',I6,13I7/)      00003510
 1920 FORMAT(I6,'-',I2,6X,16F7.1)                                   00003520
 1930 FORMAT(/' TFR   (15-49)   ',F7.1,7X,14F7.1)                   00003530
 1940 FORMAT( ' TFR* (15-44)   ',F7.1,7X,14F7.1)                    00003540
 1950 FORMAT(/' GFR   (15-49)   ',F7.1,7X,14F7.1)                   00003550
 1960 FORMAT( ' GFR* (15-44)   ',F7.1,7X,14F7.1)                    00003560
 1970 FORMAT(/' STD GFR (15-49)',F6.1,7X,14F7.1)                    00003570
 1980 FORMAT( ' STD GFR*(15-44)',F6.1,7X,14F7.1)                    00003580
 1990 FORMAT(/)                                                     00003590
 5000 FORMAT(/ 1X,2A1,1X,50A1/1X,100A1/                            00003600
     1 10X,'CENSUS YEAR-',I4,10X,'TFR=',F8.1,10X,'GFR=',F9.1)       00003610
      RETURN                                                        00003620
      END                                                           00003630
```

BIBLIOGRAPHY

Afzal, Mohammad. 1974. *The Population of Pakistan*. CICRED Monograph Series. Islamabad: Pakistan Institute of Development Economics.

Arnold, Fred, Chintana Pejaranonda, and Minja Kim Choe. 1985. *Provincial Level Fertility Estimates for Thailand, 1965–1979: An Application of the Own-Children Method*. Bangkok: National Statistical Office.

Arretx, Carmen, William Brass, Jose Alberto Magno de Carvalho, Valeria da Motta Leite, Thomas W. Merrick, Axel I. Mundigo, and Hania Zlotnik. 1983. *Levels and Recent Trends in Fertility and Mortality in Brazil*. Committee on Population and Demography, Report No. 21. Washington, D.C.: National Academy of Sciences.

Avery, Roger C. 1978. Comparing vital rates estimated from vital statistics with those estimated from own-children methods with example from Costa Rica. Paper presented at Annual Meeting of the Population Association of America, Atlanta.

Barlema, Jan, Juan Chackiel, Kenneth Hill, Mario Isaacs, and Augusto Soliz. 1985. *Fertility and Mortality in Bolivia and Guatemala*. Committee on Population and Demography, Report No. 28. Washington, D.C.: National Academy of Sciences.

Blacker, John, and William Brass. 1979. Experience of retrospective demographic enquiries to determine vital rates. In L. Moss and H. Goldstein (eds.), *The Recall Method in Social Surveys*. London: University of London Institute of Education.

Brass, William. 1975. *Methods for Estimating Fertility and Mortality from Limited and Defective Data*. Chapel Hill: International Program of Laboratories for Population Statistics, University of North Carolina.

———. 1976. Personal communication.

Chidambaram, V. C., and Zeba A. Sathar. 1984. *Age and Date Reporting*. Unpublished manuscript, World Fertility Survey, London.

Cho, Lee-Jay. 1968. Income and differentials in current fertility. *Demography* 5:198–211.

———. 1969. *Estimates of Fertility for West Malaysia*. Research Paper No. 3. Kuala Lumpur: Department of Statistics.

———. 1971a. Korea: Estimating current fertility from the 1966 census. *Studies in Family Planning* 2:74–78.

————. 1971b. On estimating annual birth rates from census data on children. In *Proceedings of the American Statistical Association, Sociological Statistics Section,* pp. 86–96.

————. 1971c. Preliminary estimates of fertility for Korea. *Population Index* 37:3–9.

————. 1973a. *The Demographic Situation in the Republic of Korea.* Papers of the East-West Population Institute, No. 29. Honolulu: East–West Center.

————. 1973b. The own-children approach to fertility estimation: An elaboration. In *International Population Conference, Liège, 1973,* Vol. 2:263–78. Liège: International Union for the Scientific Study of Population.

————. 1974. *Estimates of Current Fertility for the Republic of Korea and Its Geographical Subdivisions: 1959–1970.* Seoul: Yonsei University Press.

Cho, Lee-Jay, Fred Arnold, and Tai Hwan Kwan. 1982. *Fertility Transition in the Republic of Korea.* Washington, D.C.: National Academy of Sciences.

Cho, Lee-Jay, and Ruby Bussen. 1980. Use of own-children data for reconstruction of maternity histories. Paper presented at the International Union for the Scientific Study of Population (IUSSP) Seminar on the Analysis of Maternity Histories. London.

Cho, Lee-Jay, and Griffith Feeney. 1978. Fertility estimation by the own-children method: A methodological elaboration. Reprint Series, No. 20. Chapel Hill: International Program of Laboratories for Population Statistics, University of North Carolina.

Cho, Lee-Jay, Wilson H. Grabill, and Donald J. Bogue. 1970. *Differential Current Fertility in the United States.* Chicago: Community and Family Study Center, University of Chicago.

Cho, Lee-Jay, and Man Jun Hahm. 1968. Recent change in fertility rates of the Korean population. *Demography* 5:690–98.

Cho, Lee-Jay, Jing Qing Han, and Bo Hua Li. 1985. Application of own-children method to the household data of the 1982 National Fertility Survey of the People's Republic of China. Paper presented at the International Symposium on Analysis of the 1982 China National Fertility Survey, Beijing.

Cho, Lee-Jay, James A. Palmore, and Lyle Saunders. 1968. Recent fertility trends in West Malaysia. *Demography* 5:732–44.

Cho, Lee-Jay, and Robert D. Retherford. 1978. Own-children fertility estimates by duration since first marriage: Preliminary results for Cheju Province, Republic of Korea. *Asian and Pacific Census Forum* 5 (1):6–10.

————. 1986. Fertility transition in the Republic of Korea. Unpublished manuscript, East–West Population Institute, Honolulu.

Cho, Lee-Jay, Sam Suharto, Geoffrey McNicoll, and S. G. Made Mamas. 1976. *Perkiraan Angka Kelahiran dan Kematian di Indonesia Berdasarkan Sensus Penduduk 1971* (Estimates of fertility and mortality in Indonesia based on the 1971 Population Census). Series Sensus Penduduk 1971, SP 76-L 02. Jakarta: Biro Pusat Statistik.

————. 1980. *Population Growth in Indonesia: An Analysis of Fertility and Mortality Based on the 1971 Population Census.* Monographs of the

Center for Southeast Asian Studies, Kyoto University. Honolulu: University Press of Hawaii.

Coale, Ansley J. 1955. The population of the United States in 1950 classified by age, sex, and color—A revision of census figures. *Journal of the American Statistical Association* 50:16–54.

Coale, Ansley J., Lee-Jay Cho, and Noreen Goldman. 1980. *Estimation of Recent Trends in Fertility and Mortality in the Republic of Korea.* Washington, D.C.: National Academy of Sciences.

Coale, Ansley J., and Paul Demeny. 1966. *Regional Model Life Tables and Stable Populations.* Princeton: Princeton University Press.

———. 1983. *Regional Model Life Tables and Stable Populations.* Second edition. New York: Academic Press.

Coale, Ansley J., and Norfleet W. Rives, Jr. 1973. A statistical reconstruction of the black population of the United States 1880–1970: Estimates of true numbers by age and sex, birth rates, and total fertility. *Population Index* 39:3–36.

Coale, Ansley J., and T. James Trussell. 1974. Model fertility schedules: Variations in the age structure of childbearing in human populations. *Population Index* 40:185–258.

———. 1975. Erratum. *Population Index* 41:572.

———. 1978. Technical note: Finding the two parameters that specify a model schedule of marital fertility. *Population Index* 44:203–13.

Coale, Ansley J., and Melvin Zelnik. 1963. *New Estimates of Fertility and Population in the United States.* Princeton: Princeton University Press.

Cochran, William G. 1963. *Sampling Techniques.* New York: John Wiley.

Demeny, Paul, and Frederick C. Shorter. 1968. *Estimating Turkish Mortality, Fertility, and Age Structure: Application of Some New Techniques.* Institute of Statistics Publication No. 2. Istanbul: Istanbul University.

Engracia, Luisa T., Robert D. Retherford, Peter C. Smith, and Lee-Jay Cho. 1977. *Estimates of Fertility in the Philippines Derived by the Own-Children Method: 1960–68.* UNFPA-NCSO Population Research Project Monograph No. 9. Manila: National Census and Statistics Office.

Feeney, Griffith. 1974. A simpler matrix approach to polynomial interpolation. Honolulu: East–West Population Institute. Mimeographed.

———. 1980. Estimating infant mortality trends from child survivorship data. *Population Studies* 34:109–28.

Goldman, Noreen, Ansley J. Coale, and Maxine Weinstein. 1979. *The Quality of Data in the Nepal Fertility Survey.* Scientific Reports, No. 6. London: World Fertility Survey.

Grabill, Wilson H., and Lee-Jay Cho. 1965. Methodology for the measurement of current fertility from population data on young children. *Demography* 2:50–73.

Guzman, Jose M. 1980. *Evaluation of the Dominican Republic National Fertility Survey 1975.* Scientific Reports, No. 14. London: World Fertility Survey.

Hajnal, John. 1953. Age at marriage and proportions marrying. *Population Studies* 7:111–36.

Henry, Louis. 1961. Some data on natural fertility. *Eugenics Quarterly* 8:81–91.

Hobcraft, John, and German Rodriguez. 1982. *The Analysis of Repeat Fertility Surveys: Examples from Dominican Republic.* Scientific Reports, No. 29. London: World Fertility Survey.

Itoh, Tatsuya. 1981. Own-children fertility estimates in Japan. Paper presented at the Fertility Estimation Workshop, East–West Population Institute, Honolulu.

Jemai, H., and Susheela Singh. 1984. Question design for measurement of selected demographic events. Paper presented at the World Fertility Survey Symposium, London.

Kawasaki, Shigeru. 1985. Fertility estimation by the own-children method in Japan. Paper presented at the Tenth Population Census Conference, East–West Center, Honolulu.

Kitagawa, Evelyn M. 1955. Components of a difference between two rates. *Journal of the American Statistical Association* 50:1168–94.

Levin, Michael J., and Robert D. Retherford. 1982. The effect of alternative matching procedures on fertility estimates based on the own-children method. *Asian and Pacific Census Forum* 8 (3):11–17.

———. 1986. *Recent Fertility Trends in the South Pacific.* Papers of the East–West Population Institute, No. 101. Honolulu: East–West Center.

Little, Roderick J. A. 1982. *Sampling Errors of Fertility Rates from the WFS.* WFS Technical Bulletin No. 10. London: World Fertility Survey.

Myers, R. J. 1940. Errors and bias in the reporting of ages in census data. *Transactions of the Actuarial Society of America* 41, Part 2:395–415.

Potter, Joseph E. 1977. Problems in using birth-history analysis to estimate trends in fertility. *Population Studies* 31:335–64.

Ratnayake, Kanthi, Robert D. Retherford, and S. Sivasubramaniam. 1984. *Fertility Estimates for Sri Lanka Derived from the 1981 Census.* Matara, Sri Lanka: Department of Geography, Ruhuna University; Honolulu: East–West Population Institute, East–West Center.

Republic of Korea National Bureau of Statistics. 1984. *The Levels and Trends of Fertility for Small Geographical Areas in Korea.* Seoul.

Retherford, Robert D. 1978. Single-year computational procedures used in the own-children method of fertility estimation. *Asian and Pacific Census Newsletter* 4 (3):5–8.

Retherford, Robert D., and Iqbal Alam. 1985. *Comparison of Fertility Trends Estimated Alternatively from Birth Histories and Own Children.* Papers of the East–West Population Institute, No. 94. Honolulu: East–West Center.

Retherford, Robert D., and Neil G. Bennett. 1977. Sampling variability of own-children fertility estimates. *Demography* 14:571–80.

Retherford, Robert D., Aphichat Chamratrithirong, and Anuri Wanglee. 1980. The impact of alternative mortality assumptions on own-children estimates of fertility for Thailand. *Asian and Pacific Census Forum* 6 (3): 5–8.

Retherford, Robert D., and Lee-Jay Cho. 1978. Age–parity-specific birth rates and birth probabilities from census or survey data on own children. *Population Studies* 32:567–81.

————. 1981. Decomposition of change in the total fertility rate in the Republic of Korea, 1960–1975. *Asian and Pacific Census Forum* 7 (3):5–9.

Retherford, Robert D., Lee-Jay Cho, and Nam-Il Kim. 1983. Estimates of current fertility derived from the 1980 Census of the Republic of Korea. *Asian and Pacific Census Forum* 9 (3):12–15.

————. 1984. Census-derived estimates of fertility by duration since first marriage in the Republic of Korea. *Demography:* 537–74.

Retherford, Robert D., Minja Kim Choe, and Anuri Wanglee. 1978. An improved procedure for adjusting for omissions and age misreporting of children in the own-children method of fertility estimation. *Asian and Pacific Census Newsletter* 4 (4):5–7.

Retherford, Robert D., and G. Mujtaba Mirza. 1982. Evidence of age exaggeration in demographic estimates for Pakistan. *Population Studies* 36 (2): 257–70.

Retherford, Robert D., G. Mujtaba Mirza, Mohammad Irfan, and Iqbal Alam. 1985. Own-children estimates of fertility derived from successive censuses and surveys in Pakistan. Paper presented at the Tenth Population Census Conference, East–West Population Institute, Honolulu.

Retherford, Robert D., and Naohiro Ogawa. 1978. Decomposition of the change in the total fertility rate in the Republic of Korea, 1966–1970. *Social Biology* 25 (2):115–27.

Retherford, Robert D., Chintana Pejaranonda, Lee-Jay Cho, Aphichat Chamratrithirong, and Fred Arnold. 1979. *Own-Children Estimates of Fertility for Thailand Based on the 1970 Census.* Papers of the East–West Population Institute, No. 63. Honolulu: East–West Center.

Retherford, Robert D., and William H. Sewell. 1986. Intelligence and family size reconsidered. Paper presented at the Annual Meeting of the Population Association of America, San Francisco.

Rindfuss, Ronald R. 1976. Annual fertility rates from census data on own children: Comparisons with vital statistics data for the United States. *Demography* 13:235–49.

————. 1977. *Methodological Difficulties Encountered in Using Own-Children Data: Illustrations from the United States.* Papers of the East–West Population Institute, No. 42. Honolulu: East–West Center.

Rindfuss, Ronald R., and James A. Sweet. 1977. *Postwar Fertility Trends and Differentials in the United States.* New York: Academic Press.

Schroeder, Robert, and Robert D. Retherford. 1979. Application of the own-children method of fertility estimation to an anthropological census of a Nepalese village. *Demography India* 8:247–56.

Shryock, Henry S., and Jacob S. Siegel. 1973. *The Methods and Materials of Demography.* 2 volumes. Washington, D.C.: U.S. Bureau of the Census.

Sri Lanka Department of Census and Statistics. 1978. *Life Tables 1970–72: Sri Lanka.* Colombo.

Suharto, Sam, and Lee-Jay Cho. 1978. *Preliminary Estimates of Indonesian Fertility Based on the 1976 Intercensal Population Survey.* Papers of the East–West Population Institute, No. 52. Honolulu: East–West Center.

Supraptilah, B. 1982. *Evaluation of the Indonesian Fertility Survey 1976.* Scientific Reports, No. 38. London: World Fertility Survey.

Sweet, James A., and Ronald R. Rindfuss. 1983. Those ubiquitous fertility trends: United States, 1945–1979. *Social Biology* 30:127–39.

United States Bureau of the Census. 1947. *Differential Fertility, 1940 and 1910: Standardized Fertility Rates and Reproduction Rates.* Washington D.C.: U.S. Department of Commerce.

———. 1976. *Computer Programs for Demographic Analysis.* Washington D.C.: U.S. Department of Commerce.

United States Department of Health, Education, and Welfare. 1964. *Multiple Births: U.S. 1964.* National Center for Health Statistics Series 21, No. 14. Washington, D.C.

Wang, Weizhi. 1984. A preliminary analysis of mortality in China. *Population Research* 5:25–31. Beijing: People's University Press.

Wang, Yu, and Xiao Zhenyu. 1984. A brief account of the National One-Per-Thousand Population Fertility Survey and preliminary analysis of its data. In *Analysis on China's National One-Per-Thousand-Population Fertility Sampling Survey,* pp. 3–11. Beijing: China Population Information Centre.

Zlotnik, Hania. 1982. *Levels and Recent Trends in Fertility and Mortality in Colombia.* Committee on Population and Demography, Report No. 12. Washington, D.C.: National Academy of Sciences.

DATE DUE
